Natural Eye Care Series:

Macular Degeneration
Supporting Healthy Vision Naturally

Marc Grossman, OD, LAc and Michael Edson, LAc.

ISBN 978-1-5136-6199-5
Library of Congress Control Number: 2020907503

Printed in the United States of America
Published by Safe Goods
561 Shunpike Rd., Sheffield, MA 01257
SafeGoodsPublishing.com

TABLE OF CONTENTS

AUTHORS

Marc Grossman, O.D., L.Ac., co-founder of Natural Eye Care, Inc. is best described as a holistic eye doctor. He uses a multi-disciplinary approach using nutrition, eye exercises, lifestyle changes, and Chinese Medicine. These provide him with a wide array of tools and approaches to tackle difficult eye problems. Dr. Grossman lectures nationally on natural vision care philosophy and method and teaches workshops for health care professionals including physical therapists, chiropractors and body workers, social workers, occupational therapists and other optometrists. He is a consultant to school systems, rehabilitation centers and the U.S. Military Academy at West Point. He is co-author of the acclaimed *Natural Eye Care, Your Guide To Healthy Eyes and Healing* (published Jan. 2019), as well as *Magic Eye Beyond 3D: Improve Your Vision (Volume 6)* (2004), and *Greater Vision* (2001).

Michael Edson is a co-founder and President of Natural Eye Care, Inc. He is co-author of *Natural Eye Care: A Comprehensive Manual for Practitioners of Oriental Medicine* and *Natural Eye Care: Your Guide to Healthy Vision and Healing*, 2019. Michael Edson's latest book is *Natural Parkinson's Support: Your Guide to Preventing & Managing Parkinson's* (2020). His upcoming book, *Natural Brain Support: Ways to Help Prevent and Treat Dementia and Alzheimer's Naturally* will be published in 2020.

PREFACE

Natural Eye Care Series: Macular Degeneration offers a unique approach to supporting healthy vision from early childhood to mature age, with the understanding that healthy vision relies on overall health and emotional health. Filled with wisdom and insight of both ancient and modern-day healing methods, this book integrates a wide range of alternative therapies as they apply to health of the macula.

This book will help you make sensible, researched, and clinically based decisions to support macular health with recommendations that include Western herbs, nutritional supplements, Chinese medicine, and additional therapies. You will learn about the underlying causes and be given tools and techniques to develop your own eye health strategies. If a particular problem, cluster of symptoms, or changes in vision occur we recommend you consult your eye doctor.

Natural Eye Care Series: Macular Degeneration shows you how to become an active participant in your own vision care. The primary goal of this book is to offer a practical approach, based on the underlying philosophy that emphasizes prevention and support. In doing so, we celebrate the healing power within all of us and the mind/body's inherent potential for self-healing.

Many eye care professionals annually give stronger and stronger prescriptions that help weaken the eyes instead of eye exercises and lifestyle recommendations to help strengthen vision. Something is wrong with this picture. Diet, exercise, lifestyle, and targeted supplements should be a critical part of the discussion of how to maintain healthy vision, even with specific eye conditions such as macular degeneration. The peer-reviewed research is abundant in demonstrating these alternatives.

This guide will educate readers about their vision difficulties, explain prevention strategies, and also explore ways to help preserve vision for those with vision disorders. It will enable the individual to be a more informed consumer when it comes to vision care. Medication and surgery may sometimes be necessary or even appropriate treatment strategy, but nutrition and lifestyle choices always play an essential role in helping support healthy vision.

Doctors in China have reached out to the West to borrow the modern medicine we can offer. We in the West can, in turn, benefit from the ancient wisdom of the East. By combining the medical approaches of the East and West, along with other alternative health modalities, we may be able to achieve better health with less cost and greater success in helping patients preserve vision.

Natural Eye Care Series: Macular Degeneration is dedicated to the belief that a common ground can be created in which the strengths of modern-day Western medicine are united with the preventive approach of other healing modalities.

MACULAR DEGENERATION

Macular degeneration (AMD) is the leading cause of irreversible blindness, and it is the leading cause of vision loss among people over 60.[1] It is also known as age-related macular degeneration (ARMD). By the year 2020, an estimated 7.5 million Americans will suffer significant vision loss due to this disease. In 2010, 2.5% of white adults, age 50 and older, had AMD. By comparison, AMD affected 0.9% each of Blacks, Hispanics, and people of other races. The risk of AMD increases with age. The disease is most common among older white Americans, affecting more than 14% of white Americans age 80 and older.[2] Although there is no effective conventional treatment yet, natural remedies can go a long way to help prevent this disorder from progressing to the point of vision loss.

WHAT IS MACULAR DEGENERATION?

Macular degeneration is the slow deterioration of cells in the macula, a tiny yellowish area near the center of the retina where vision is most acute. This deterioration affects central vision, the vision used for reading, writing, driving, and identifying faces. With macular degeneration, straight lines become crooked, distinct shapes are blurry, lines become wavy, and a fog forms in the center of vision. Peripheral vision, however, is not typically affected.

If AMD is found first in one eye, the other eye tends to follow the same progression. This is because the nutrient deficiencies and other system-wide problems would exist in both eyes, but manifest in one eye before the other.

The two most common types of macular degeneration are the dry and wet type. Most people with macular degeneration have the **dry type**, in which small yellow spots called "drusen" form underneath the macula. The drusen slowly break down the cells in the macula, causing distorted vision. In approximately 10–15% of cases, dry macular degeneration can progress to the second, more severe type called wet macular degeneration. In the **wet type** of macular degeneration, choroidal neovascularization occurs. This is a process in which abnormal blood vessels begin to grow toward the macula. These new vessels often leak blood, further deteriorating the macula, and causing rapid and severe vision loss if not treated.

There is a great deal of peer review research showing that the likelihood of the onset of AMD can be significantly reduced through healthy lifestyle choices such as diet,[3] [4] [5] regular exercise,[6] no smoking,[7] [8] avoidance of heavy drinking[9] (moderate drinking of wine may have a beneficial effect),[10] management of chronic stress,[11] avoidance of excess weight,[12] control of blood pressure[13] and high cholesterol,[14] and supplementation with targeted nutrients such as lutein, zeaxanthin, and omega-3 fatty acids (such as fish oil or DHA from algae).

Even when advanced AMD has developed, healthy lifestyle choices and targeted supplementation can still play a major role in slowing down and stabilizing the AMD. But lost vision, due to retinal cells no longer living, cannot at this time be regenerated, though excellent research such as with stem cells and the regeneration of lost retinal cells is underway. Keep in mind that patients can sometimes experience improved vision as retinal cells that are not active may still be living but are low functioning. These cells can be stimulated and helped to be more active through diet, exercise, and targeted supplementation.

THE RETINA

Retinal Layers
The retina consists of four different layers:

1. Outer neural layer containing nerve cells and blood vessels

2. Photoreceptor layer, a single layer containing the light sensing rods and cones
3. Pigmented retinal epithelium (RPE), with the Bruch's membrane separating the RPE from the 4th (choroid) layer
4. Choroid layer, consisting of connective tissue and very fine capillaries (choriocapillaries), that carry nutrients and oxygen to the cellular layers above them

The RPE's role is to nourish the fragile nerve tissue of the retina and maintain its health by providing blood and nutrients to the photoreceptor cells, getting rid of dead cells, secreting hormones, and

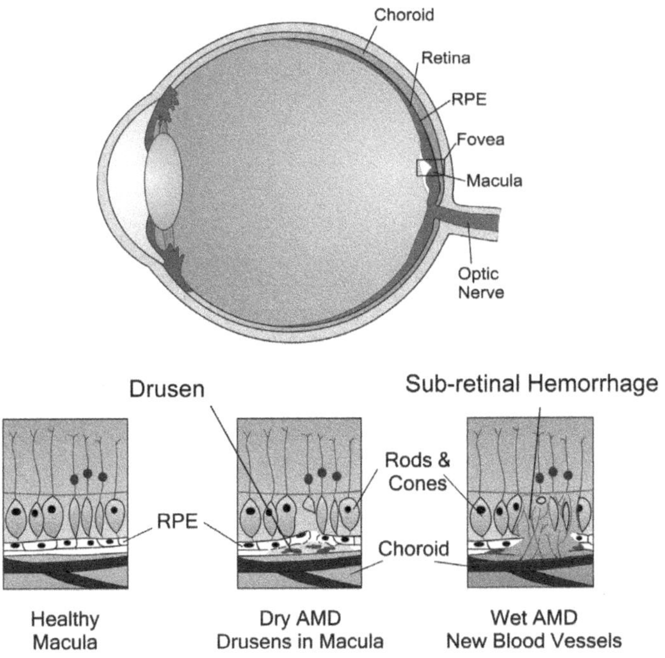

modulating immune factors. It closely interacts with photoreceptors in the maintenance of visual function.

The choroid layer contains most of the eyeball's blood vessels. It is also the layer prone to bacterial and secondary infections. If not treated, abnormal blood vessel growth can readily develop, resulting in sight impairment or eventually, total vision loss.

The Macula

The macula is located at the center of the retina where focused vision takes place. The remainder of the retina, located at the margins or periphery, is more responsible for low light vision.

The macula contains two areas of unusually high concentrations of cones, which are the photoreceptors responsible for color vision, fine detail, and central vision. There is a slightly depressed area in the center of the macula called the fovea where there are no retinal cells, only photoreceptors, approximately 199,000–300,000 cones per square millimeter. At the center of the fovea is the foveola. Here too there are only cones, no rods.

The gradual breakdown of these cells in the macula results in damage to, or loss of, your central vision. Because the macula provides focus in the center of vision, where your vision sharpness is most acute, such deterioration reduces the ability to read and to recognize faces, two important tasks that require central vision.

TYPES OF MACULAR DEGENERATION

Dry Macular Degeneration

Dry AMD (about 90% of cases) is also known as geographic atrophy. The atrophy results from the inability of the retina to reabsorb natural waste created in the retina in the process of passing light from the photoreceptor cells to the optic nerve (and other normal physiological activity). This further results in a slow deposit of the waste (drusen) onto the retina, which over time, can result in loss of healthy vision.

DRUSEN

Drusen are thought to be comprised of waste proteins and lipids (oily material) that begin to accumulate due to poor circulation and waste flushing in the eye. Antioxidants are important for the normal waste-clearing process and have the potential for reducing drusen in the eyes.[15] [16] [17] The drusen slowly crowd, distort, or break the cells in the macula, leading to deterioration, and resulting in blurred vision. Because the drusen also include immune-system regulating molecules, it is thought that they are part of the immune system.[18]

EARLY DIAGNOSIS

AMD has few symptoms in the early stages, so it is important to have your eyes examined regularly. If there are drusen on the retina, the initial diagnosis may not be dry AMD until the eye doctor determines that the number of drusen is increasing. For people who have early (dry) AMD in both eyes, about 10–15% will develop wet AMD in at least one eye after 10 years.

Wet Macular Degeneration

Untreated dry macular degeneration can worsen to "wet" macular degeneration. New blood vessels begin to form near the macula (choroidal neovascularization). These new vessels can leak fluid and blood, which may lead to swelling and damage of the macula. Unlike the more gradual course of dry AMD, wet AMD damage can be rapid and severe. It is possible to have both geographic atrophy (dry) and neovascular (wet) AMD in the same eye, and either condition can appear first. A retinal exam can identify whether there is leakage or bleeding in the retina or only drusen. Research shows that a healthy diet and taking targeted supplements can significantly reduce the onset of neovascularization.[19] [20] [21]

Stargardt Disease

Stargardt disease affects about 1 in 10,000 children in the U.S. Although the disease starts before age 20, you may not notice vision loss until age 30–40. It is a genetic form of macular degeneration where patients need to avoid supplements with vitamins that contain vitamin A and beta-carotene, foods high in vitamin A and beta-carotene, and certain carotenoids that can be converted to vitamin A in the body.[22]

Myopic Macular Degeneration

Myopic macular degeneration typically occurs in those people who are very nearsighted. In these cases, there is an extreme elongation of the eyeball, which causes stretching of the retina and can result in tears in the macula and bleeding beneath the retina. Over time, this can cause cells in the macula at the center of the retina to atrophy or die, causing a blind spot in the center of the visual field. In some cases, this form of macular degeneration can turn into wet AMD. People who are very nearsighted who generally require glasses of -6 diopters or more, are at risk for myopic macular degeneration. The risk is higher as myopia becomes worse than -10 diopters.

PATHOLOGY OF MACULAR DEGENERATION

The development and progression of macular degeneration rests upon the occurrence of the following pathological changes in the eye:

Oxidative stress is the imbalance between free radicals and protective antioxidants. The retina is especially vulnerable to stress from free radicals. Inability of the retina tissue to have enough oxygen leads to deterioration of the pigmented layer, which protects the retina from UV and blue-light damage.[23] Antioxidants can significantly reduce the effects of oxidation stress.[24]

Angiogenesis, the development of new and extra blood vessels, is caused by insufficient oxygen in the retina. The tightly packed retinal formation gets crowded by these additional blood vessels, and the retina becomes distorted. Targeted nutrients can inhibit such new and unwanted blood-vessel growth.[25]

Apoptosis, (cell death) is a natural phenomenon in the body, by which worn and damaged tissue is removed and replaced. However, in the retina, excessive cell death is closely tied to oxidative stress.[26] Reducing oxidative stress through nutrients such as antioxidants and enzymes can reduce apoptosis.[27]

Inflammatory response is a process where the body rushes nutrients and oxygen-carrying blood to an injured location. The body always attempts to rescue tissue from cell injury due to oxidative stress through this response. However, this natural response can also result in vision damage over time, due to scar tissue and bleeding in the retina (angiogenesis).[28]

SIGNS AND SYMPTOMS

- Lines look distorted or wavy. Try the Amsler test on page 55. In more developed AMD, the Amsler grid can look quite distorted.
- Shapes look blurred, fuzzy, or hazy in central vision.
- Colors appear dimmer and less distinct.
- Words are hard to read because they are blurred.
- Blank or dark areas hide the center area of your vision.
- The center of vision looks foggy or cloudy.

CAUSES AND RISK FACTORS

AMD that is diagnosed from childhood into adulthood but before the age of 50 is typically considered to be the result of genetics. One study determined that there was a 12-fold increase in the risk of getting macular degeneration if you have a sibling with AMD.[29] The risk factor was considered high if you have a parent with AMD.[30]

Heredity is a risk factor. People who have a family history of AMD are more at risk to develop it. The field of epigenetics shows that, even though one may have a genetic disposition for AMD (or any other health condition), environmental factors, including early childhood nurturing and lifestyle choices, can play a significant role in whether these genes become active or not.[31]

Free radicals can damage the eyes. They are formed when the blue and ultraviolet sunlight passes through the crystalline lens of the eye. Free radicals are also byproducts of our bodies' natural metabolic processes. These chemicals are highly reactive and cause oxidation; the result is destabilization of healthy macula cells.[32]

Phototoxicity is caused by exposure to blue and ultraviolet (UV) radiation, both of which adversely affect the functioning of retinal pigment epithelium (RPE) cells. RPE cells are susceptible to cell death induced by ultraviolet B (UVB) radiation. Exposure to sunlight without protective sunglasses is a risk factor for AMD.

Nutrition and diet can play an important role. Research has proven that elder people with poor diets are more prone to developing AMD. Micronutrient supplementation enhances antioxidant defense and healthy eyes, and it might prevent, retard, and modify vision loss.[33] People with AMD are often deficient in a number of nutrients that are essential to eye health: antioxidants, carotenoids, essential fatty acids, enzymes, minerals, and amino acids.[34]

Hypertension. People with high blood pressure are more likely to develop AMD than those with normal blood pressure.[35]

Smoking increases the risk of AMD by 200–300%. Smoking, chronic fatigue, and a weakened immune system hasten damage from free radicals.[36] [37]

Systemic inflammation, indicated by high levels of C-reactive protein, has been tied to increased macular degeneration risk.[38]

High homocysteine levels may contribute to AMD.[39] [40]

Women[41] and **diabetics**[42] are more at risk to develop AMD.

Prescription and over-the-counter drugs can damage the retina.[43] These include:

- Plaquenil (hydroxychloroquine sulfate), often prescribed for rheumatoid arthritis and found to cause permanent damage to the retina
- Catapres (clonidine hydrochloride is the generic name) for high blood pressure
- Chloridine (Catapres) for high blood pressure
- NSAIDS (non-steroidal, anti-inflammatory drugs) include ibuprofen, aspirin, ketoprofen, flurbiprofen, and naproxen sodium; side effects from their regular use include retinal hemorrhages

RELATED CONDITIONS

Poor circulation in the eye is a contributing factor to many eye conditions and is a side effect of diabetes.[44] Elevated homocysteine levels have been associated not only with macular degeneration but also glaucoma, diabetic retinopathy, optic neuropathy, and ocular complications from Behcet disease. [45] Also related are macular pucker or epiretinal membrane (where a thin layer of tissue grows over the retina), and retinitis pigmentosa (a degenerative disorder of the photoreceptor cells of the retina).

CONVENTIONAL TREATMENT

No effective conventional treatment currently exists for dry macular degeneration. However, since the AREDS studies in 2001, 2003, and clarification in 2013, some eye doctors are beginning to recognize the value of nutritional supplementation.

Injections

Wet macular degeneration is typically treated with injections of Lucentis, Avestin, or Eylea. These drugs have antiangiogenic properties, meaning they help prevent the growth of new blood vessels, while drying up existing blood vessels that leak. The injections are typically necessary on an ongoing basis, depending on the severity and history of bleeding. Over the long run, they do not necessarily prevent vision loss; however, they can be essential for helping to slow down the progression of wet AMD. Moreover, these drugs are not designed to address the underlying problem, which in most cases is the inability of the body to deliver essential nutrients to the retina, and/or lack of critical nutrients, and/or inability of the eyes to naturally eliminate waste materials that are generated on an ongoing basis in the retina. Ultimately, our short-term goal is to stabilize the AMD, and the long-term goal is to maintain healthy vision and prevent additional vision loss. Drugs can have potentially serious side effects, so the benefits of using them should be evaluated with your eye doctor and your family.

Surgery

Laser surgery (photodynamic therapy) may be an alternative option to injections if the eye doctor determines that the injections may be ineffective or contraindicated for the patient. Your eye doctor will be able to provide guidance on the best therapy for you. Laser surgery accurately targets and seals leaking blood vessels through the injection of a form of ink into the blood stream, which gets absorbed at a much higher rate by leaking blood vessels than healthy ones. Then a non-thermal or "cold" laser is directed at the abnormal blood vessels in the eye for approximately 90 seconds. The laser activates the dye, which destroys the abnormal blood vessels and spares the normal retina and normal blood vessels.

Genetic Testing

FOR AMD RISK

Though genetic testing is available now to help determine one's risk of getting AMD, there has been some controversy among eye-care professionals as to whether genetic testing should be done for at-risk patients with certain genetic polymorphisms that have discrete genetic variations: CFH and ARMS2.

FOR ZINC HYPER-IMMUNE RESPONSE

Sometimes certain supplements can cause problems for specific genetic variations of AMD. It has been suggested that certain patients actually do worse with zinc supplementation. In 2015, the recommendations from Bascom Palmer stated that there was not enough evidence to recommend routine genetic testing when considering supplementation. Dr. Stuart Richer, lead researcher in the last lutein antioxidant supplementation trial, recommends that the use of lower amounts of zinc (less than 50mg daily) is as effective as higher doses. He also recommends that genetic testing be offered to monocular-vision patients (where our two eyes have two views; we see near and far distance differently) to avoid the possibility of a zinc hyper-immune response, which is a possibility for 1 out of 7 high-risk AMD patients.

COMPLEMENTARY APPROACH

As always, prevention is the best medicine. Since less than 1% of people with macular degeneration have progressed to the point of legal blindness, most are in a position to benefit greatly from preventive measures, particularly at the earlier stages of the disease.

Taking targeted supplements and establishing healthy lifestyle habits are still helpful at any stage of AMD, keeping in mind that the preservation of vision and potential level of vision improvement is based on the vision level the patient has at the time of incorporating complementary approaches.

Proper diet, nutritional supplementation, and lifestyle improvements, including regular exercise and stress management, are fundamental to any prevention program, or adjunct to treatment for macular degeneration. Macular degeneration is a difficult disease to control, and we need to incorporate the best of current knowledge in nutritional support and supplementation.

NUTRIENTS

★ ★ ★ ★ ESSENTIAL

Abundant research has brought the carotenoids into the mainstream of vision care.[46] [47] The landmark studies that came to the attention of many conventional eye doctors were the Age-Related Eye Disease Studies (AREDS).[48] There were two studies: AREDS (2001), AREDS2 (2006), and the AREDS update in 2013, which laid out protocols for macular degeneration (AMD) treatment that include carotenoids, vitamins, and omega-3 fatty acids.[49]

Carotenoids lutein, zeaxanthin, meso-zeaxanthin, and astaxanthin are essential. Xanthophylls absorb short wavelength blue, violet, and ultraviolet light which penetrate all the way to the back of the retina. The shorter a wavelength, the greater the energy it possesses, and so these blue to ultraviolet wavelengths have the potential of damaging the retina, resulting in oxidative stress to the retina and its center, the macula.

> Researchers found that a **moderate dose of 13.3mg combined carotenoids**, comprised of 83% lutein (11mg), 10% zeaxanthin (1.33mg), and 7% meso-zeaxanthin (.93mg), was more effective than higher doses in enhancing **macular pigment**, even though higher doses were reflected in serum blood levels.[1]

★ ★ ★ ★ **Lutein.** 6mg–20mg per day. Lutein mostly accumulates in the periphery of the retina, but also in the macula which is responsible for detailed vision. The macula is yellow because of the yellow color of lutein and zeaxanthin; it is able to absorb oxidizing blue, violet, and ultraviolet light, acting as a sort of internal pair of sunglasses that protect the eyes against damage from sunlight.[50] [51] [52] [53] [54]

AMD. Lutein lessens the risk of damage from age-related macular degeneration. Diets rich in lutein reduce AMD risk by 57%.[55] Treatment with lutein helps thicken the protective pigmented layer of the retina;[56] retinas with AMD have 30% less lutein than healthy retinas.[57]

Lutein is even more effective when coupled with the carotenoids, zeaxanthin, and meso-zeaxanthin. Lutein also reduces the risk of progression (by 25–30%) of the dry (early) form of macular degeneration into the more severe (wet) form, choroidal neovascularization.[58]

- **Antioxidant.** The retina is constantly exposed to oxygen and light, resulting in oxidative stress and phototoxic stress. Lutein[59] does not have a direct role in the process of sight. Rather, its powerful antioxidant ability protects the macula by absorbing damaging blue, violet, and ultraviolet light[60] that causes stress and free-radical activity. It further accomplishes this by supporting macular pigment thickness,[61] the eye's defense against damaging UV and blue light.
- **Inflammation.** Lutein is more than merely a filter for the sun's UV radiation. A 2012 research study found that it modulates inflammation in the eye, such as that manifested in laser-induced choroidal neovascularization (wet macular degeneration).[62]

Sources. The best source of lutein is kale and then spinach. Other good sources include: turnip greens, summer squash, Brussels sprouts, orange foods (such as corn, pumpkin, paprika, yellow-fleshed fruits), pecans, and avocado.

Lutein is also available through enriched eggs. A small study found that lutein from enriched eggs was absorbed more easily than lutein from spinach or supplements.[63] In addition, the lutein that comes from red and orange foods supports macular pigment density more than that from spinach or supplements.[64]

Caution. People with cystic fibrosis may not very well absorb lutein from supplements.

★★★★ Meso-zeaxanthin. 10mg. This carotenoid is found to help central vision in the retina. Studies show that supplementing with meso-zeaxanthin helps protect central vision for those with AMD. It is the most powerful of the three antioxidants in the macula, but is most effective in combination with lutein and zeaxanthin.[65] Levels of all three carotenoids (lutein, zeaxanthin, and meso-zeaxanthin), when increased in the blood, increase macular pigment density.[66] [67]

AMD. A number of studies show that supplementing daily with meso-zeaxanthin, along with lutein and zeaxanthin, significantly increases macular pigment[68] (found to be compromised in those with AMD).

Sources. It is found in microalgae and sea creatures that consume the algae, such as trout, salmon, shellfish, and krill. It is found in the skin of trout, sardines, and salmon.

★★★★ Zeaxanthin. 2mg–12mg per day.[69] Zeaxanthin is concentrated in the macula where it fights oxidative stress. Along with lutein, it comprises the macular pigment, a yellow pigment that absorbs blue light. It improves central vision function in a number of ways.70 Its color-filter capacity protects photoreceptor cells (cones) from light-originated free-radical damage.

AMD. A number of studies found that high intake of zeaxanthin lowers the risk of dry AMD advancing to the more serious form, wet AMD.[71] It does so by increasing the density of the macular pigment.[72] Zeaxanthin is even more effective than lutein in protecting against oxidative stress from ultraviolet light exposure.[73] It improves vision in elderly patients with early AMD, according to both eye charts and reports of better night vision.[74]

- **Antioxidant**. Zeaxanthin has similar properties to lutein; it is a retinal pigment and potent antioxidant.
- **Glare recovery.** One of the diagnostic tests for macular problems (as distinct from optic nerve problems) is the glare recovery test in which the subject is exposed to bright light, such as the eye doctor's ophthalmoscope; the recovery time is measured according to how long it takes for visual acuity to return. Zeaxanthin, lutein, and meso-zeaxanthin make up most of the macular pigment and are essential for good recovery from glare.[75]

Both lutein and zeaxanthin supplements are best taken separately from beta-carotene supplements because of competition for absorption. Lutein and zeaxanthin need fat to absorb well, so take them with food or a small amount of oil.

Sources. The best source of zeaxanthin is kale and then spinach. It is found in orange and red foods such as saffron, orange peppers, paprika and paprika peppers, goji berry, corn, oranges, and tangerines. Other vegetables such as collards, mustard greens, romaine lettuce, broccoli, kiwi fruit, peas, and chard contain a lot of the zeaxanthin.

★★★★ Omega-3 fatty acids. 2,000mg–3,000mg per day. Omega-3 fatty acids are a specific type of essential fatty acid known to reduce inflammation and lower the risk of chronic diseases. Omega-3 fatty acids, found in fish, are a primary component of retinal photoreceptors and of the myelin sheath that surrounds nerve fibers in the eye.

They are so essential to the retina that when omega-3 levels begin to fall, the retina begins to recycle DHA within the eye. The typical American diet is deficient in omega-3 fatty acids but has too much omega-6s (from vegetable oils and refined grains).

There are three types of omega-3 fatty acids: alpha-linolenic acid (ALA), which is found in plant oils; eicosapentaenoic acid (EPA) used primarily in the brain and retina, and docosahexaenoic acid (DHA) used primarily in the heart and circulatory system; the latter two are found in fish oils.[76] EPA and DHA are not naturally present in the body; we can synthesize them from ALA, but this ability declines with age. Therefore, it is important to get adequate EPA and DHA from other sources.

The primary omega-3 fatty acids, DHA and EPA, may protect the retina through expression of genes, retinal cell differentiation, and survival. There has been extensive research about these two omega-3's and much less about alpha-linolenic acid (ALA). It is likely that the three have very specific and independent roles in protecting against disease.[77]

AMD. DHA has been found to have antioxidative, anti-inflammatory, antiapoptotic, and anti-angiogenic (limiting growth of new blood vessels) effects.[78] [79] [80] [81] [82] [83] [84] [85] While it is known that a low-fat diet (10% from fat) lessens AMD risk, it has been found that omega-3 fatty acids and olive oil further reduce AMD risk. [86] Eighty-five percent of AMD patients over age 70 experienced improved vision after four weeks of supplemental omega-3s.[87] Other reports, such as a meta-analysis of more than 270 studies and papers,[88] a longitudinal study of over 1,800 people over 12 years,[89] and a large 10-year study evaluating the diets of nearly 40,000 women confirmed these findings.[90]

- **Antioxidant.** A derivative of DHA protects retinal pigment epithelial cells from oxidative stress.[91] Unlike the effect of

DHA in other parts of the body such as the liver, it does not appear to be subject to lipid oxidation in the retina.[92]

- **Inflammation.** DHA reduces inflammation [93] in retinal microcapillaries[94] and in the retina, changing potent inflammatory agents to less powerful ones.[95] Omega-3s reduce neuroinflammation.[96]

- **Neovascularization.** EPA and DHA have the capacity to regulate formation of blood vessels, which is important with respect to the advanced form of AMD, choroidal neovascularization.[97] [98] They are able to encourage immune cell movement toward the site of extraneous formations of blood vessels that distort vision. The results indicate promising potential for omega-3 as a nutritional therapy that includes other conditions involving both inflammation and neovascularization.[99]

- **Neuroprotection.** Omega-3 fatty acids are essential for nerve conduction in the retina and for retinal blood flow. Omega-3 DHA is present in large amounts in retinal epithelial cells, acting towards neuroprotection; this understanding presents possibilities for future therapies.[100]

Sources.
- EPA. Cold-water fish, especially mackerel, lake trout, sardines, tuna, and salmon. Also, halibut, river trout, catfish, cod, red snapper, and tuna packed in water.
- DHA. Some microalgae, anchovies, salmon, herring, mackerel, tuna, and halibut. Also, liver, fish oil, and eggs from grass fed poultry.
- ALA. Flaxseed, flaxseed oil, canola oil, pumpkin seeds, pumpkin seed oil, tofu, perilla seed oil, walnuts, walnut oil, and chia seeds.

✭✭✭✭ Resveratrol. 150mg–175mg per day, (trans-resveratrol is a well absorbed form). It appears to target multiple age-related issues such as mitochondrial dysfunction, inflammation, angiogenesis,[101] and oxidative stress.

AMD. Resveratrol and its components protect against development of lipofuscin, damaged cells that accumulate in the Bruch's membrane and which generate fatty yellow drusen, characteristic of AMD.[102]

- **Antioxidant.** Resveratrol's antioxidant action protects the cardiovascular system, helps maintain biochemical balance, and protects neurons from injury or degeneration.[103] [104] [105] [106] [107]

- **Inflammation.** Resveratrol's anti-inflammatory capacity may help protect microcirculation in the eye.[108] By reducing inflammation, it helps maintain biochemical balance and protects the nervous system.[109]

Sources. Grape skins, grapeseed extract, sprouted peanuts, and in lesser amounts cocoa powder, and dark chocolate. It is present in a variety of berries including blueberry, bilberry, currant, and cranberry. Heating and cooking these berries reduce the amount of available resveratrol.[110]

Note: Grapeseed extract (300mg daily) is another proanthocyanidin with functions similar to resveratrol.[111] [112] [113]

✭✭✭✭ Saffron. Saffron is better known as a kitchen spice that lends yellow color and a delicate flavor to many dishes. It can have wonderful results for eye problems.

AMD. Studies have shown that saffron helps protect photoreceptor cells from damage and supports healthy circulation in the retina.[114] [115] [116] [117] [118] [119] Patients given saffron supplementation show improved macular pigment thickness and retinal function,[120] as well as improved electroretinogram results, indicating improved flicker sensitivity in early macular degeneration, suggesting that improvements may extend beyond the benefits of antioxidant support.[121] [122]

Sources. Saffron is available as a supplement but made-at-home saffron tea made from hot water and at least 10 strands of good quality saffron is great tasting and soothing.

★★★★ Vitamin C (buffered and ascorbated). 2,000-3,000mg recommended per day.

Vitamin C is a necessary ingredient for many enzyme processes in the body, supporting injury healing and blood vessel integrity. It is helpful for a wide range of eye conditions. It is a powerful antioxidant and helps remove oxidized waste material in the body.[123] [124] [125] [126] [127] After the adrenal glands, the second highest concentration of vitamin C is in the eye. Vitamin C enhances the absorption of lutein, which is one of the most important vision antioxidants.[128]

AMD. The AREDS studies established that vitamin C was one of the nutrients helpful in preventing dry AMD and preventing development into wet AMD (choroidal neovascularization). [129] It's best to supplement with an ascorbated vitamin C, buffered with bioflavonoids and/or minerals.

Sources. The highest levels of vitamin C are found in rose hips, raw sweet red peppers, oranges, grapefruit, and green peppers. Other good sources are kiwi fruit, broccoli, strawberries, tomatoes, cantaloupe, and cabbage. Vitamin C is destroyed by heat and prolonged storage.

★★★★ Vitamin D3. 2,000 IU–5,000 IU per day.

Fat-soluble vitamin D is actually a group of vitamins that perform a number of essential functions, including proper absorption of magnesium and calcium.[130] Vitamin D synthesis comes primarily from a process involving the sun. Our skin contains a biochemical precursor to vitamin D, a form of cholesterol called 7-dehydrocholesterol. When the skin is exposed to UV light rays, cholecalciferol is created, and a process begins that passes through the liver, then to the kidneys where it is converted into calcitriol, vitamin D.[131]

AMD. Low levels of vitamin D3 in the body can be connected to an increase in the presence of macular degeneration[132] and supplementing with D may lower risk,[133] especially in women younger than age 75. Vitamin D supports the health of the retinal microvascular system.[134]

Sources. Sunlight is a great source of D. Foods include fatty fish, vitamin D fortified foods, and smaller amounts of beef liver, cheese, and egg yolks. Vitamin D3 is a more readily absorbed form of D.

Caution. Get exposure to the sun in only short spurts (10-15 minutes), avoiding sunburn. Skin pigmentation and climate are factors determining when the body reaches a saturation point and stops producing vitamin D.

★★★★ Vitamin E. Vitamin E is made up of four tocopherols and four tocotrienols, but alpha tocopherol is the main vitamin E form in the body.

AMD. In a study of patients and controls over age 60, researchers found a marked connection between incidence of AMD and low blood plasma levels of zinc and vitamin E. In addition, they found that the lower the level of vitamin E, the greater the severity of AMD.[135] The AREDS studies of 2001, 2003, and update in 2013, confirmed the helpfulness of vitamin E.[136]

- **Antioxidant.** Vitamin E is fat-soluble and an antioxidant, and it scavenges free radicals formed from oxidation of lipids (fats).[137]

- **Immunity and inflammation**. It affects the expression and activity of immune and inflammatory cells and to enhance dilation of blood vessels.[138]

Sources. The best source of vitamin E is wheat germ. Other good sources include sunflower seeds, almonds and other nuts, spinach, and broccoli.

Note. Vitamin E as a supplement is most effective when taken in the mixed tocopherol form.

★★★ VERY IMPORTANT

★★★ Astaxanthin. 6mg–12mg per day. Astaxanthin is another powerful antioxidant that is effective in protecting against damage from light [139] [140] and protecting the photoreceptors [141] through its antioxidative capacity and through its activation of a by-product, Nrf2.[142]

One unique quality is its ability to cross the blood/brain barrier,[143] which means that it has the capacity to deliver antioxidants directly to the eyes, the brain, and the nervous system. This explains its presence in the retina.

AMD. Astaxanthin, for antioxidant effect, is added to many of the nutritional supplements used in AMD patients.[144] Reviews[145] [146] of previous and ongoing research point to the wide range of benefits of this potent antioxidant, including excellent tolerability and safety factors. Astaxanthin lowers levels of free radicals in people who are smokers or overweight; it blocks oxidative damage to DNA, acts as an anti-inflammatory agent, supports tuberculin immunity, lowers triglycerides, increases blood flow and good HDL cholesterol, supports brain functioning with improved cognition and nerve stem cell growth, improves visual acuity,[147] reproductive health, and more.[148]

- **Antioxidant.** Astaxanthin destroys free radicals, and wards off their constant attack towards all parts of the body.[149] When tested against a wide variety of ROS and RNS (nitrogen-reactive species) molecules, astaxanthin was one of the most effective in free radical scavenging. Its antioxidant ability is ten times more powerful than beta-carotene,[150] lutein, or zeaxanthin, and from 60–500 times stronger than vitamin E.[151] [152] It must be taken through food or in supplement form since it is not made by the body.

- **Inflammation.** Astaxanthin is also a powerful anti-inflammatory agent and pain reliever. Because inflammation is at the root of many eye conditions, this ability to reduce inflammation is extremely beneficial. It is able to block COX-2 enzymes, which cause the pain and inflammation behind various forms of arthritis.[153]

- **Eye fatigue.** In a number of different studies, researchers found that astaxanthin was useful in reducing fatigue, sore dry eyes, blurry vision, and recovery from intense visual stimulation.[154] [155] In computer users, astaxanthin was found to significantly improve accommodation amplitude, which refers to the ability of the eye to change focus as distances change.[156] [157] [158] [159] [160]

Sources. Sources include red yeast Phaffiarhodozyma (used in Asian cooking), salmon, shrimp, trout, and other pink seafood that eat the red algae Haematococcus.

⭐⭐⭐ Bilberry. 120mg–180mg per day. Bilberry is a small wild shrub growing in North America and northern Europe. It is famous for its value for vision health.[161] [162] [163] [164]

AMD. Bilberry is helpful for macular degeneration because it protects the retina against oxidative stress that results from the activity of free radicals.[165] It is an effective neuroprotector.[166]

- **Antioxidant**. Antioxidant[167] anthocyanosides are the active components of bilberry. They help improve microcirculation of tiny blood vessels [168] [169] [170] [171] [172] and therefore, improve the delivery of oxygen to the eyes. They accomplish this by improving rhythmic changes in the diameter of blood vessels[173] [174] in the eye's vascular system, as well as in the entire body. They help repair and protect retinal tissue,[175] [176] and generally support a healthy retina by supporting levels of antioxidants in the blood serum.[177]
- **Inflammation.** Bilberry is also rich in tannins, which are astringent in nature and have anti-inflammatory properties.

★★★ Curcumin. Curcumin is a powerful anti-inflammatory and antioxidant agent with many beneficial effects. It is the primary ingredient of turmeric, a bright yellow spice used to add color and flavor to curry, mustard, and more. It is a relative of ginger.

AMD. Vascular endothelial growth factor (VEGF) is a protein that, among other functions, regulates cell death and has been the subject of extensive research. Anti-VEGF therapy is a common treatment for wet macular degeneration. Curcumin has been shown to inhibit VEGF and cell death and is of great interest to researchers.[178] Curcumin has been found to have a protective effect against cell damage in human retinal pigment cells caused by blue light, because it protects retinal pigment epithelial cells against oxidation, which is caused by free radicals.[179] Consequently curcuminoids may have potential in AMD treatment.[180] [181]

- **Inflammation.** Curcumin is known for its ability to fight inflammation, which is a key component of many health conditions.[182]

Sources. Turmeric (curcuma longa), mango ginger (curcuma amadaRoxb), and curry powder.

★★★ Ginkgo biloba. 120mg per day. Ginkgo has been used for many centuries for eye and central nervous system problems. It is a selective cerebrovascular dilator[183] that seems to increase circulation and blood flow to the back of the eye and the body.

Ginkgo's beneficial properties come from its flavonoid constituents. Ginkgo contains quercetin, kaempferol, and isorhamnetin, which are known as flavonoid glycosides (meaning that they include a molecule of sugar). This is important because flavonoids such as quercetin are known to be difficult to absorb, but the presence of sugar improves their bioavailability.[184]

AMD. Ginkgo may help improve impaired vision due to dry age-related macular degeneration, by improving normal function and tone of blood vessels[185] [186] [187] and by reducing oxidative stress on the retinal pigment epithelial cells.[188] [189]

★★★ Glutathione (GSH), reduced. 500mg–900mg per day. This potent antioxidant has been shown to help protect retinal cells from damage. Best to take sublingually, as it is not well absorbed through capsules or tablets.[190] Sublingual doses are typically lower, as they are absorbed 5–10 times more efficiently than capsules or tablets.

AMD. Low levels of glutathione are observed in macular degeneration patients. Early macular degeneration patients have high levels of oxidized glutathione (glutathione disulfide), which is a biomarker for AMD.[191]

- **Antioxidant.** Glutathione is one of the "super" antioxidants because it is capable of stabilizing the full spectrum of free radicals. It is used throughout the body and is considered one of the essential anti-aging nutrients. The amount of glutathione in blood plasma is considered an overall indicator of the body's antioxidant defense system.[192]
- **Mitochondrial support.** It is involved in the control of mitochondrial membrane permeability and therefore helps protect against premature cell death.[193] It is not generally considered an essential nutrient since the body is capable of synthesizing it from a number of amino acids, including cysteine, glutamic acid, and glycine. However, cysteine is somewhat rare in foods so that the amount of cysteine in the body determines how much glutathione can be produced.

Sources. Since glutathione is poorly absorbed when taken directly in pill or capsule form, we recommend taking a formula that is either sublingual or submucosal and contains additional nutrients to help the liver manufacture additional glutathione.

★★★ Taurine. 750mg–1,000mg per day. Taurine is another potent antioxidant found in the retina. It is essential in helping the eyes eliminate waste and enhancing the rods and cones within the retina, which serve as visual receptors.[194] [195] [196] Taurine is critical for nerve health and is responsible for clearing away and regenerating old tissue. It is especially important for the health of the eye and of the inner ear.

AMD. Low levels of taurine are associated with instances of AMD[197] and macular dystrophies.[198] Taurine protects against ultraviolet radiation, acts as an antioxidant to protect cells, helps move nutrients across cell membrane barriers, and helps remove debris and toxins from the system.[199]

Taurine protects against retinal degeneration. Research has shown that when taurine is removed from food, animals develop retinal degeneration; when taurine is replaced, the degeneration reverses.[200] [201] [202] [203]

Sources. Highest levels of taurine are found in shellfish, especially clams, scallops, and mussels, as well as dark poultry meat. Lower amounts of taurine are found in cheese.

★★★ Lycopene. 3mg per day. Lycopene is bright red in color and found in red fruits and vegetables, but not all red foods contain lycopene. In order for it to be absorbed by the body, it has to combine with fats, and it is best utilized when cooked in the presence of fat.[204] It may be that supplements are more effectively absorbed than food, especially if the food source is raw.[205]

AMD. People with the lowest serum levels of lycopene, the most abundant carotenoid in the serum, were twice as likely to have macular degeneration when compared to those having the highest levels.[206]

- **Antioxidant.** Lycopene is the most powerful antioxidant in the carotene family. Researchers describe it as the "most efficient biological carotenoid singlet-oxygen quencher."[207] Some researchers feel that its benefit comes indirectly from the lycopenoids produced by lycopene, rather than its own antioxidant capacity.[208]
- **Inflammation**. Lycopene is protective against nerve inflammation[209] caused by oxidative stress. Free radicals cause oxidative stress, which in turn damages and inflames healthy nerve cells.

Sources. Guavas have the most lycopene, followed by red watermelon and tomatoes, especially cooked or sun-dried. Other vegetables include sweet red peppers, asparagus, red cabbage, and carrots. Fruits include papaya, pink grapefruit, and mango.

Caution. If taken with anticoagulant drugs, lycopene can increase the risk of bleeding. It also interacts with medications for blood pressure, the immune system, sunlight sensitivity, and some gastrointestinal drugs. Some people are allergic to lycopene.

★★★ Melatonin. Melatonin is a hormone that occurs naturally in the body; production increases as darkness falls and declines in the morning. Reduced levels of melatonin are linked to increased risk of AMD along with other problems such as poor sleep.

AMD. A research study showed that a combination of melatonin (3mg), zinc (8.7mg), and selenium (50 mcg), taken before bedtime, helped stabilize AMD with some remarkable improvement in the fundus of the eye after taking the combination for 6 months.[210] [211] In lab animals melatonin protected against a complication of AMD known as non-exudative AMD (caused by atrophy or detachment of the pigmented RPE layer of the retina).[212] It is thought that melatonin's ability to reduce mitochondrial dysfunction makes it useful as a treatment for AMD.[213]

Sources. These foods either contain melatonin or are helpful in converting serotonin to melatonin. Sour cherries, corn, asparagus, tomatoes, pomegranate, olives, grapes, broccoli, cucumber, rice, barley, oats, and nuts (not too much) such as walnuts, peanuts, sunflower seeds, and flaxseed.

★★ IMPORTANT

★★ **Quercetin.** Quercetin is a flavanol that protects the eye from chronic solar radiation exposure. The flavanols are aromatic, colorless compounds that occur in plants. They are found as glycosides, which means they are bound to a sugar molecule.

In addition, quercetin reduces inflammation. It is being investigated for use in helping reduce allergy-related eye symptoms. It functions in a synergistic manner with vitamin E and taurine. Quercetin helps protect fine capillaries in the retina from deterioration and leaking. Both quercetin and rutin are important for a healthy macula.

AMD. Quercetin is helpful through its antioxidant capacity to protect retinal pigment from oxidative stress that is caused by solar radiation.[214] Quercetin also inhibits formation of extra blood vessels, and as well, it improves blood flow in the choroid layer of the retina.[215]

Sources. Quercetin is highest in lingonberries. It is also found in dark red or blue fruit, such as cranberries and blueberries, as well as in black and green tea, capers, apples, red grapes, citrus, broccoli, and leafy-green vegetables. It is also in tomatoes. Interestingly, organically grown tomatoes have 79% more quercetin than chemically grown tomatoes.[216]

Caution. Supplemental quercetin may be contraindicated for quinolone antibiotics, such as fluoroquinolone, because it binds to the bacteria, but researchers don't understand whether this is a problem.[217] It is also identified as having potentially interfering interactions with taxol/paclitaxel used to treat some types of cancer.[218]

★★ **Zinc.** This mineral is not itself an antioxidant but has some antioxidant characteristics. Zinc is part of the molecular structure of more than 100 enzymes and is involved in the synthesis of many amino acids. It has roles in RNA and DNA metabolism, cell death, gene expression, and neuron and synapse activity, but it can also be a neurotoxin in the brain.[219] It helps heal injuries, supports the immune system, and supports the functioning of many enzymes.

Zinc plays a vital role in bringing vitamin A from the liver to the retina in order to produce melanin, a protective pigment in the eyes. It helps bind the protective pigment layer of the retina to the underlying tissue. Zinc is found in high concentrations in the eye, especially the retina, its underlying tissues, and choroid (the vascular tissue layer lying under the retina).[220]

AMD. The AREDS studies demonstrated that zinc is helpful for macular degeneration,[221] slowing progression of the condition and protecting retinal health.

Sources. Highest concentrations are in red meat, oysters, crab, and lobster. Vegetable sources depend on the soil quality; organic products are probably the best sources: wheat germ, wheat bran, seeds (sunflower and pumpkin), beans, nuts (especially almonds), whole grains, chicken, and turkey.

Caution. Zinc restricts copper, so if you are taking zinc you should also take copper as well in a 15:1 zinc to copper ratio. Consult your health care professional.

★ HELPFUL

★ **Green tea.** 500mg–750mg per day. The major bioflavonoid catechins found in green tea are epicatechins, antioxidants which inhibit ocular neovascularization and protect the microcapillaries of the retinal pigment epithelium by reducing neovascularization, a complication of AMD.[222] [223] [224]

Through studies with lab animals, researchers have found that green tea catechins are passed from the digestive system into the tissue of the eye.[225] Green tea contains a variety of other phytonutrients that support its value.

- **Antioxidant protection**. Tea catechins protect against oxidative stress due to chemical damage; they also protect the mitochondria.[226] [227]
- **Retinal support**. Green tea epigallocatechin protects the retinas of lab animals from the oxidative damage of hydrogen peroxide[228] and from UVB light damage. This UV light protective effect seems to have to do with the ability of cells to resist degradation when exposed to UV light.[229]

Sources. In addition to green tea, catechins are especially abundant in cocoa and chocolate, but you should limit the quantity. They are found in abundance in dark plums and broad beans, such as fava beans. They are also found in pecans, red wine, strawberries, apples, peaches, and black grapes.

★ CoQ10. 100mg–200mg per day. Study findings strongly suggest that an appropriate combination of acetyl-L-carnitine, omega-3 fatty acids, and coenzyme Q10, which affect mitochondrial lipid metabolism, may improve and subsequently stabilize visual functions; it may also improve fundus alterations in patients affected by early AMD and helps reduce drusen.[230] [231]

Co-enzyme Q10 is a vitamin-like antioxidant that is produced by the body and is also available in food. It supports mitochondria processes in the retina.[232] Mitochondria are the cellular energy producers that support all cellular activity. Depletion or deficiency of CoQ10 is thus a deficiency of one of the fundamental needs of the cell in every part of the body. Other nutrients such as acetyl-l-carnitine, omega-3 fatty acids, vitamin E, and alpha-lipoic acid enhance CoQ10 functioning.

AMD. CoQ10, combined with acetyl-L-carnitine or omega-3 fatty acids, supports retinal functioning more than either of those nutrients alone. In general, compounds that affect mitochondrial fat metabolism appear to improve and stabilize vision, and even improve vision in patients with early-stage AMD.[233] In combination with acetyl-L-carnitine, omega-3s, and vitamin E, it improves the retinal pigment cell tissue function[234] and reduces the drusen-covered area of the retina.[235]

- **Retinal disease.** Not only does CoQ10 play an essential role in mitochondria processes, but it also protects fats, proteins, and DNA from oxidative stress. The reviewers note its value in treating AMD and glaucoma and propose that it could be effective for other retinal conditions.[236]

Sources. Meats and fish are among the best sources of CoQ10. Other good food sources include nuts, seeds, broccoli, cauliflower, oranges, and other fruit.

✭ Goji berries. A study found that daily supplementation with a milk and goji formulation increased the levels of zeaxanthin in the blood and increased protection from additional drusen formulation or loss of pigmentation.[237]

✭ Selenium. 200mcg per day. Selenium is an essential trace element needed to synthesize enzymes, such as the antioxidant glutathione that is essential to healthy vision. AMD patients have low blood plasma levels of selenium.[238] [239]

Sources. Brazil nuts, seafood, whole grains, seeds, meat, poultry, and mushrooms. Other good sources include garlic, onions, broccoli, cabbage, and sunflower seeds.

✵ **L-methionine.** The essential amino acid L-methionine is synthesized in the body as part of the metabolism of proteins, which is an intermediate step to the creation of cysteine, carnitine, and taurine—all critical to eye health.

Its conversion to cysteine requires adequate levels of B vitamins. As a part of certain cell functions, it contributes a molecule to the process, and is "repaid" that molecule from vitamin B12 or folic acid. However, when the body is deficient in those nutrients, this repayment (remethylation) does not occur, and homocysteine remains. Over time, high levels of homocysteine build up, which have been connected to a number of vision and health conditions.

AMD. There are connections between high levels of homocysteine and advanced macular degeneration,[240] [241] other retinal conditions, and photoreceptor problems.[242]

Sources. This nutrient is found in egg whites, fish, poultry, and crustaceans. In smaller quantities it is found in seaweed, sesame seed, and cottage cheese.

✵ **Magnesium.** One of the most abundant elements in the body, magnesium is critical for the metabolism of many other minerals, of nitric oxide, and of many enzymes in order to maintain equilibrium within cells. Absorption of magnesium, in turn, depends upon many other factors including magnesium in the diet, selenium, parathyroid hormone, and vitamins B6 and D. Excess fat interferes with magnesium functioning. In addition, too many alcoholic beverages, salt, sugary sodas, coffee, women's menstruation issues, sweating, stress, certain drugs, and parasites can decrease the levels of magnesium.[243]

AMD. Many researchers have observed that patients with macular degeneration are low in magnesium (along with lack of enough vitamin E, B6, folic acid, and zinc).[244] Poor retinal microcirculation, preventing adequate supply of nutrients, is one factor in AMD that is affected by magnesium levels.

Sources. Dry roasted almonds, spinach, cashews, soymilk, beans, and avocado, as well as wheat germ, fish, and also various leafy-green vegetables.

Caution. If you are taking antibiotics, do not take magnesium because it interferes with the effectiveness of the antibiotics.

★ Rutin. Rutin (containing one molecule of quercetin) is an anti-oxidant and an excellent free-radical fighter.

AMD. Rutin combats inflammation and oxidative stress involved in the development of macular degeneration. Furthermore, research has indicated that rutin reduces leakage from tiny retina blood vessels and combats inflammation.[245]

Sources. Capers have the highest concentration of rutin, seven times as much as black olives, and nine times as much as buckwheat. It is found in large amounts in raw asparagus, black tea, and black and red raspberries. To a lesser degree, it is found in citrus fruits, mulberries, cranberries, peaches, cherries, white grapefruit, pears, grapes, red onions, onions and garlic, green cabbage, spinach, and kale.

★ Triphala. This ayurvedic formulation is a compound of three dried and powdered fruits (haritaki, bibhitaki, and amalaki), with both nourishing and detoxifying properties. It is rich in polyphenols, flavonoids, and vitamin C.[246] It is antifungal, protects cells from harmful agents,[247] and is an anti-inflammatory antioxidant.[248]

AMD. Triphala is useful in reducing inflammation and growth of new blood vessels (in wet AMD) by inhibiting production of a cytokine which is implicated in both diabetic retinopathy and neovascularization in the choroid and retina.[249] In addition, individually, amalaka[250] and haritaki,[251] [252] have been found to reduce damage caused by macular degeneration.

★ Vitamin B6.

This B vitamin assists in a number of enzyme activities, especially in amino acid synthesis, glucose metabolism, and fat metabolism. Along with folic acid and B12, B6 is responsible for converting homocysteine to cysteine (needed for glutathione production).

AMD. Most macular degeneration patients tend to be deficient in vitamin B6, and so it is generally included in formulations for vision health. In people with more than three AMD risk factors or cardiovascular disease, researchers found that folic acid, B6, and B12 combined could reduce the risk of AMD.[253]

Sources. Vegetables contain the most stable form of B6, pyridoxine. Good sources include avocado, wheat bran, organ meats, molasses, milk, and eggs.

★ Vitamin B12.

The body builds up large reserves of vitamin B12 over time, and so people who lack B12 in their diets may not experience serious symptoms of deficiency for many years. It is critical to proper functioning of brain and nerve cells. Supplementation may reduce eyesight deterioration from glaucoma by supporting myelin sheath stability (the fatty layer surrounding nerve cells).

Along with folic acid and B6, B12 is responsible for converting homocysteine to cysteine. Low levels of B12 are linked to high levels of homocysteine. High homocysteine levels are associated with many vision conditions, including glaucoma, diabetic retinopathy, and optic neuropathy.

AMD. There have been contradictory reports as to whether B12 is helpful for AMD. A review of eleven relevant studies (about 2,000 people) found that AMD is linked to high levels of homocysteine and low levels of B12.[254] Whether B12 or the other B vitamins are helpful for AMD is still under evaluation.

Sources. The best sources of B12 are clams and beef liver, followed by fish, milk, cheese, and eggs. Only fortified grains contain B12.

Note. Methylcobalamin, the natural form of B12 in nature, is easily absorbed and utilized by the body. This is the only form of vitamin B12 one should supplement with. The cyanocobalamin form of B12 is completely synthetic and contains trace amounts of cyanide, which, although not considered toxic in the amounts taken in, is a toxin that has to be eliminated from the body if in excess.

Caution for Vegetarian/vegans. Vegetarians often have vitamin B12 deficiency and those on vegan diets must supplement with B12.

Diet

★★★★ Vision Diet. Follow a strong alkaline diet to reduce overall inflammation in the body, as chronic inflammation has been identified as a contributing factor to macular degeneration.[255] Both local and systemic inflammatory processes contribute to the development and progression of AMD.[256] For some people, chronic inflammation may be related to leaky gut syndrome, so if applicable, an anti-inflammatory diet should be adopted.

Many research studies have shown that diet has a significant effect on health of the macula. Unfortunately, once a person has macular degeneration, a healthy diet is not enough to prevent this disease from worsening, so other interventions are needed, which may include conventional as well as targeted supplementation, diet, exercise, and lifestyle changes.

★★★★ Leafy greens. Make sure your diet includes plenty of fresh, preferably organic, dark leafy greens. These vegetables are rich in carotenoids, which help plants absorb light energy for use in photosynthesis, and they deactivate free radicals, meaning they have antioxidant properties and are helpful for the entire body. Two of these carotenoids, lutein and zeaxanthin, are of particular importance to eye health. So, even if you don't like vegetables such as collard greens, kale, Swiss chard, and spinach, you can add them to soups, puree them in green drinks, juice them with other fruits and vegetables, or add them to other greens in salads. The nutrients found in these healthy vegetables lower the risk of developing macular degeneration.[257]

★★★★ Antioxidants. Diets high in antioxidants help protect AMD patients from vision loss and play two critical roles: first, they significantly reduce the risk of AMD onset, and second, they help protect AMD patients from vision loss.[258] [259] [260] [261] A diet high in antioxidants includes fruits, particularly colored fruit such as berries that are lower in sugar, and vegetables, particularly leafy-green vegetables and colored vegetables such as red, green, and yellow peppers.

★★★★ Take **omega-3 fatty acids** from oily fish, such as wild caught salmon and sardines. These reduce the risk of developing AMD.[262] [263] [264] [265] [266] [267]

★★★ **Reduce sugars.** Reduce or eliminate all types of refined sugars (particularly white sugar, but also fructose, sucrose, fruit juice concentrates, maltose, dextrose, glucose, and refined carbohydrates). This includes "natural" drinks that contain a lot of sugar, including all fruit juices. Even milk sugar, lactose, found in all dairy products, can contribute to macular degeneration. Sugar contributes to overall body inflammation and poor circulation throughout the body and eyes. In one study, those in the highest one-fifth of the dietary glycemic index, (a system that ranks foods, based on their blood-sugar effect on a scale from 1 to 100), had more than a 40% increased risk of significant macular degeneration than those in the lowest one-fifth.[268]

★★★ **Artificial sweeteners.** Avoid all artificial sweeteners as they have been shown to be neurotoxic.[269] [270]

★★★ **Water.** Drink 8 eight-ounce glasses of water per day (preferably filtered or purified). This is optimally taken as a four-ounce glass of water every half-hour, to equal 16 four-ounce glasses. Our bloodstream can only effectively handle about four ounces at any one time. When you drink more than four ounces at a time, it means more work for the kidneys to filter water that hasn't had a chance to travel through the lymph system and clean body tissues. Adequate water intake helps maintain the flow of nutrients to the lens and release wastes and toxins from tissues.

Spring water without chlorine or fluoride is the best. Drinking filtered water may remove needed minerals. Adding back a full complement of electrolytes will help prevent mineral deficiency that exacerbates dehydration.[271] Sip water throughout the day, and do not rely on feeling thirsty before drinking.[272] At the point you feel thirsty, your body is already dehydrated. Neurological changes start occurring when there is a 2% drop in total body water. Also, certain eye diseases, as well as general health diseases, have been associated with dehydration.[273]

★★ Reduce fats. Favor a diet moderate in fats, as high levels can disturb the proper balance of gut bacteria essential for proper digestion and overall health.[274] [275] Keep polyunsaturated fats to a minimum,[276] and eliminate any trans-fatty acids in your diet, which can increase cholesterol levels, free-radical activity, and inflammation, all of which affect the eyes' blood vessels.[277] [278]

★★ Limit refined carbohydrates.[279] Refined carbohydrates are those foods that have been processed, particularly related to many of the white foods including white pasta, rice, flour, bread, and white sugar.

★★ Dairy. Limit or eliminate dairy products. For some people, regular consumption of dairy products can exacerbate eye problems by causing sinus congestion, which can impair lymph and blood drainage from the area around the eyes. When lymph and blood cannot flow in and out of the eyes, nutrients cannot efficiently reach the eyes, and toxins and metabolic wastes are not eliminated as well.

Many people are lactose intolerant to some degree, so you may want to avoid dairy for at least one month to experience the effects and observe the differences in your body and eyes. As a general rule reducing or eliminating dairy from your diet has many benefits.

Regular milk contains two types of beta-casein protein: A1 and A2. A2 milk, marketed under that brand name, contains no A1 protein. There is controversy as to whether A1 milk is more harmful than A2, but the evidence is not conclusive. It may be that the type of feed, chemicals, antibiotics, and pasteurization/homogenization cause problems rather than casein type.

If you want to consume dairy, you can try organic products from A2 cows. Alternatively, you can switch to goat milk since milk from goats does not carry the A1 gene, or at the very least, obtain fresh, raw milk from local farmers for the freshest product. In general, changes in lifestyle related to healthier vision and the taking of targeted supplements will start making a difference right away, though it may take three to six months before maximum benefits begin.

LIFESTYLE

The following are additional measures for the prevention or treatment of macular degeneration:

★★★★ Sunglasses. Wear outside in bright sunlight. They should be 100% UVA and UVB blocking lenses with wrap-around sides. Amber or brown lenses are the most effective colors for neutralizing the blue-light spectrum, which is as potentially damaging as UVA and UVB light. Wear sunglasses along with a three-inch brimmed hat.

★★★★ Exercise regularly. Exercise positively affects the health of our bodies in many ways, including increased circulation.

★★★★ Avoid blue light. Reduce exposure to artificial blue light from computer screens, cell phones, LED, and fluorescent lighting. Even low levels of blue-light exposure (400-470nm) may induce photoreceptor and retinal-pigment-epithelial cell damage.[280] Light-induced damage also increases with age, due to a decrease in protective enzymes such as superoxide dismutase (SOD). Artificial blue-light exposure appears to be more damaging at night than during the day.[281] Blue light permanently damages retinal cells, and once lost, they cannot regenerate. Replace all fluorescent and LED lighting with incandescent bulbs. Other lighting options include beeswax candles and Himalayan salt lamps. There are blue-light-blocking glasses (ex: Blutech lenses or complete protection BP1550 tints) that can be worn while on the computer, as well as blue-light-blocking programs that can be downloaded to your computer and phone.

★★★ Microcurrent stimulation. Daily sessions at home. The MCS 100ile unit is the most researched unit used for retinal health related to AMD. According to researchers the modality is both effective and safe, and it has a positive benefit for AMD patients.[282] [283] [284] [285] [286] [287] [288] [289] Microcurrent Stimulation is used to support retina health by stimulating energy production (ATP) in the retina, improving circulation & reduce waste build-up. Patches are placed directly over the eyes.

MicroCurrent Stimulation (MCS) 100ile is an enhanced adaptation of an FDA approved therapy used by anesthesiologists, orthopedic surgeons, plastic surgeons and rehabilitative specialists to promote the healing of wounds and transplanted tissues as well as to treat pain. Seven studies have been done to date supporting the benefits of using specific microcurrent settings and frequencies for retinal issues.

Note. Usage may vary depending on the type of microcurrent unit you use, so check with your healthcare practitioner to get proper instructions. If you have a history of retinal bleeding, do not use MCS without checking with your eye doctor. Contraindications include having a pacemaker or a history of epilepsy.

★★★ Do not smoke. Smoking increases the risk of AMD onset by two to three times.[290]

★★ Avoid aspirin. Aspirin thins the blood, so some doctors recommend it for improving blood flow to the retina; but several studies have shown that aspirin actually can cause macular degeneration through retinal hemorrhages.[291] Therefore, try to avoid aspirin, particularly if there is a history of macular degeneration in your family.

★★ Avoid EMF. Avoid, or severely restrict, sources of non-native electromagnetic frequencies (nn-EMF). Higher EMF exposure leads to hypoxia, dehydration, and inflammation.[292] [293] [294] [295] Turn off all WiFi signals at night such as the internet modem, wireless printers, cell phones, computers, etc. When talking, don't put your cell phone next to your head. Use the speaker instead.

★★ Touch the earth. Ground yourself as much as possible by allowing any part of your body (bare skin) to directly touch the ground (by walking barefooted or by gardening without gloves). This allows you access to the earth's abundant negative ions that can protect us from free-radical induced inflammation and cellular damage. Grounding connects you to the earth's magnetic field and can protect your body from man-made EMF, UV light, and cosmic radiation.[296]

★★ Eye Exercises. Both eye exercises and physical exercises are extremely important in the treatment and prevention of eye conditions. Exercise raises oxygen levels in the cells and increases lymph and blood circulation. This increased circulation revitalizes the organs and glands and speeds up detoxification of the body. I recommend that you gently build up to aerobic exercise for a minimum of 20 minutes per day, four days a week.

For our spirit and emotions, it is good to take some time for yourself everyday whether it be a walk in the woods, yoga class, meditation, prayer, etc. We tend to get engrossed in the daily routines of our life without taking quality time out for ourselves. We recommend you try the following eye exercises: A free book on how to do these exercises is mentioned in the Resource Directory at the end of this book.

- Palming
- Eye massage
- Near and far
- Hot dog

Natural Eye Care: Macular Degeneration

There are a number of acupuncture/acupressure points around the eyes (basically around the orbits of the eyes which are the bones that surround the eyeballs). The points shown above are some of the major local eye points.

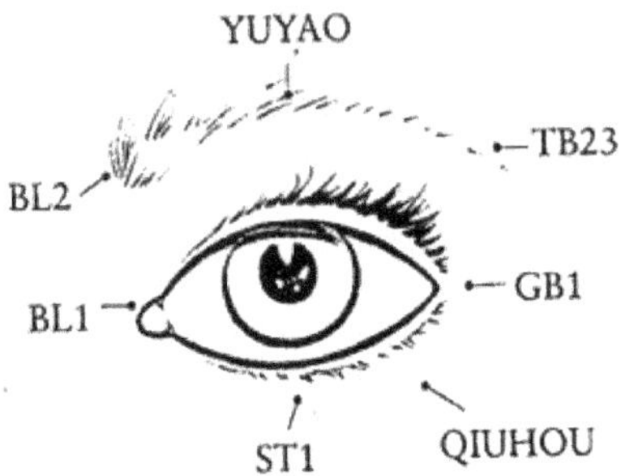

GENTLY massage each acupuncture point around the orbit of the eye, starting with B1-1 and massaging each point as you go up and outward. Each point should be massaged for approximately 5-10 seconds. You can massage both eyes at the same time. You can do this massage as often as you like over the course of the day. You may find that each point feels different in terms of sensitivity.

Keep BREATHING as you massage. Deep breathing helps the cells of your eyes receive the oxygen they need for healing. Practice long, slow abdominal breathing while massaging the acupressure points.

Caution: If you are pregnant, consult a trained acupuncturist before treating yourself. Do not massage on an area if it has a scar, burn or infection.

OTHER MODALITIES

Chinese Medicine

In Chinese medicine, the Liver "opens to the eyes" and is the primary meridian for supporting overall flow of energy and circulation through the eyes. The Kidney meridian nourishes the blood to the eyes, and the Spleen meridian also nourishes the blood while helping to prevent fluids from leaking from blood vessels. Other meridians may also be out of balance that can affect eye health, so an evaluation by an acupuncturist can best determine where the out-of-balances are and offer the optimal treatment strategy.

Chinese Medicine Patent Formulas

- **Xiao yao san** is a classic Liver tonic used in Chinese medicine that supports healthy circulation and the free flow of energy in the eyes as well as throughout the body.
- **Ming mu di juang wan** is another classic formula used in Chinese medicine for eye health. It helps nourish the Kidneys and Liver. It is known to help with blurriness of vision, tearing against wind, and conjunctive congestion with pain and swelling.
- **Celosia 10** was designed for retinal disorders based on formulas described in Chinese research reports.

Homeopathic Formulas

Homeopathic preparations, such as macula homeopathic pellets (by Natural Ophthalmics), support macula health. Follow directions on the bottle.

Essential Oils

Carrot seed improves the eyes by protecting against macular degeneration, detoxifying blood vessels, toning the liver, relieving stress and anxiety, and providing many nourishing vitamins and minerals.

Frankincense has been around since antiquity, a sacred plant that can be helpful in showing us our visual blind spots. Frankincense tells us to "open up that third eye."

Note: Keep essences away from the mouth, eyes, and mucous membranes; if a few drops get in one of these sensitive areas it may be uncomfortable for 15–30 minutes, but not harmful. You can lessen discomfort by adding a pure oil like olive or coconut oil to neutralize the irritating effect. For the eye area, dab a few drops around the outside of the eye. Do not put the neutralizing oil in the eye.

Combine ¼ cup of avocado oil with ¼ cup of calendula-infused oil. Slowly add 5 drops each of the essential oils. Then close the bottle and shake well; apply 4 drops of this mixture on your clean face. Massage in gentle circular motions. Leave overnight.

Chelation Therapy

At least one case study has been published where chelation therapy was helpful for macular degeneration caused by blockage in the choroid capillaries.[297]

EDTA, a synthetic amino acid, is commonly used as part of chelation therapy, as it may directly remove calcium found in fatty plaques that block arteries, thus breaking up the plaques. In one study, the researchers found a clinically modest, but statistically significant, benefit of chelation therapy for cardiovascular events.[298] In another study, calcification in coronary artery disease was reversed by EDTA-tetracycline long-term chemotherapy.[299]

Caution. Chelation therapy removes minerals from the body, resulting in deficiencies. Your doctor will need to monitor mineral and kidney function.

Hyperbaric Oxygen Therapy

Hyperbaric oxygen therapy may be effective in the treatment of both wet and dry macular degeneration. The treatment involves inhalation of 100% total oxygen in a chamber where atmospheric pressure is increased and controlled, according to the Hyperbaric Medical Society.[300] [301] There was one report of exacerbation of macular edema linked to this therapy.[302]

Ozone Therapy

Two small clinical studies suggest that ozone therapy may trigger defenses against damage to photoreceptors by improving blood flow and various biomarkers indicative of dry AMD resulting in improved vision sharpness.[303]

Intravenous (IV) Nutrient Therapy

IV nutrient therapy is a technique in which vitamins and other nutrients are delivered directly into the bloodstream in an IV solution, flooding the body's cells with higher levels of the nutrients than they would get from ingesting them. IV nutrient therapy can help both wet and dry AMD by delivering essential nutrients needed by the retina to help maintain healthy vision.

In his August 2010 issue of *Bottom Line Natural Healing*, Mark Stengler, a licensed naturopathic medical doctor, discusses intravenous nutrient therapy for macular degeneration. Although no clinical studies have been done, some anecdotal results have been impressive, for example, seeing more clearly after one ninety-minute treatment.[304]

Juicing

Juicing provides a concentrated source of nutrients and antioxidants and is particularly important for those people with health conditions, or even healthy people on the go that do not have the time to consistently eat a healthy diet. We recommend using only organic foods for juicing when possible.

Making freshly juiced drinks of mostly organic fruit and vegetables is a critical part of the process of healing your eyes and body. It can take only several minutes for nutrients from fresh juice to be utilized by your body. And once they are ingested, they are carried through the blood stream to all parts of your body including your eyes.

There is ample research for almost every eye and health condition that demonstrates that diets high in fruits and vegetables are critical to good health and reduce the risk of disease. Fruit and vegetables contain more protein than you might think. Vegetables such as green beans, corn, artichoke, watercress and the cabbage family (broccoli, cauliflower, brussels sprouts, etc.). have the most protein of the vegetables.

Carotenoids and bioflavonoids, for example, are phytonutrients known as phytochemicals. These are chemical compounds that exist only in fruits and vegetables and when you consume them, they help protect your health and vision. For example, lutein is found in yellow fruits and vegetables and is also in the macula of the eye, where it acts as an potent antioxidant and internal sunscreen, protecting the most sensitive part of the eye from blue, violet, and ultra violet light. Use at least four of the recommended foods below to make juice.

- Use broccoli, green and red bell pepper, raspberries, apples, copious amounts of dark leafy greens, and carrots.
- You can add favorite fruits and vegetables. Limit use of carrots, beets, and fruits due to their high-sugar content.
- Try to use room temperature vegetables and fruit.
- Do not add ice or very cold liquids since cold foods and liquids will eventually extinguish the stomach's digestive fire.
- Do not juice as often during the cooler months of the year, and instead, switch to vegetable soups or stews.

ON THE HORIZON

Ultra-fast lasers deliver gene therapy to macular degeneration patients. By using ultrafast near-infrared lasers, researchers at the University of Texas at Arlington (UTA) provide hope for eye patients suffering from photo-degenerative ailments. The platform is an improvement from current therapies that mostly slow down, or stop, degeneration, but they do not repair the damaged parts of the retina.

Epigenetic therapy integrates genetic based therapy, bio-identical hormones, and nutrition to help the body naturally repair itself at the cellular level, and it may reduce the number of injections currently needed for many with wet AMD.[305] [306]

Stem cell research has found that the cells comprising both dental pulp and the retina develop from certain stem cells. It may be possible to "re-program" these cells, thereby coaxing them into becoming retina cells. There are many safety concerns, but it is a promising avenue of exploration.[307]

Implantation of a tiny telescope for end stage AMD patients involves using micro-optical technology to magnify images, which would normally be seen in one's "straight ahead" or central vision. The telescope is smaller than a pea and uses micro-optical technology to magnify images, which are projected onto the healthy portion of the retina not affected by the disease, making it possible for patients to see or discern the central vision object of interest. This procedure is performed on an outpatient basis.

Early diagnosis. There is a simple test, currently being researched, called AdaptDx, that may be available to assess retinal function and diagnose early macular degeneration.

Vitamin E. A study published in 2018 found that blue light changes and damages a signaling biochemical, phosphatidylinositol 4,5 bisphosphate (PIP2), causing cell death; alpha-tocopherol appears to reduce that change.[308]

Amsler Grid

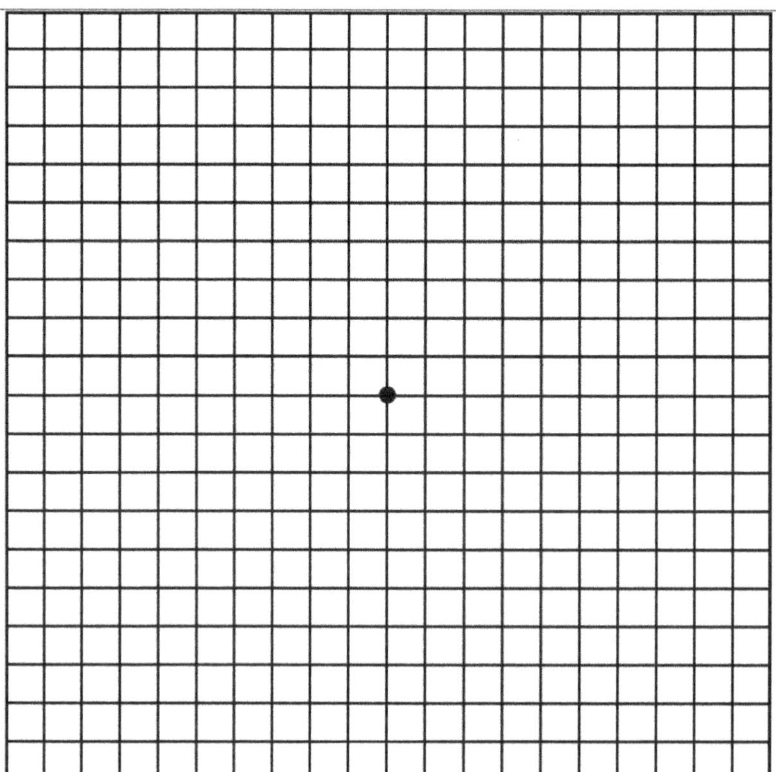

Instructions

- Test your vision with adequate lighting.
- If you normally wear reading glasses or bifocals for near work, put them on to view the grid.
- Measure (or have someone else measure) a distance of approximately 16 inches from your eyes to the screen.
- Cover your left eye, but do not close it or press on it. With your right eye, stare directly at the spot in the center of the grid, and do not look away from this spot.

(cont'd next page)

As you notice the horizontal and vertical lines in your periphery. Ask yourself the following questions as you check each eye separately: Are any of the lines:

- wavy,
- missing,
- blurry, or
- discolored?

Repeat the test with your other eye.

RESOURCES

Supplements for eye health. Natural Eye Care, New Paltz, NY www.naturaleyecare.com, email info@naturaleyecare.com, phone: 845-475-4158

Sample products:

- **Advanced Eye and Vision Support Formula** is a whole food, organic, GMO free eye formula for retinal and overall eye health.
- **Dr. Grossman's Meso Plus Formula with Astaxanthin** with mesozeaxanthin supports central vision.
- **Krill Oil or Omegagenics Fish Oil** (or a high-quality fish oil) is essential for healthy vision and overall health.
- **Vitamin D3** is shown to support overall vision and boost immunity
- **Saffron** (optimized) is shown to support healthy circulation to the retina and helps protect photoreceptor cells from damage
- **Taurine extract** used in the retina for helping eliminate waste and is a potent antioxidant.
- **Eye exercise booklet** mentioned on page 47 is available at no charge on the website: NaturalEyeCare.com
- **electroBlast™ electrolyte concentrate.** Add to purified water to restore full-spectrum ionic trace minerals to your drink.

Note: Most of these nutrients are also shown to be healthy for the brain, heart, and overall health.

Phone consultations and record review contact:
Dr. Marc Grossman, email: drgrossman2020@gmail.com

End Notes

---

[1] Macular Degeneration Partnership. AMD is the leading cause of vision loss of people over 60. Retrieved Oct 15 2016 from http://www.amd.org/what-is-amd.html.

[2] National Eye Institute. Age-Related Macular Degeneration (AMD). Retrieved Oct 31 2017 from https://nei.nih.gov/eyedata/amd.

[3] (2014). Micronutrient supplementation enhances antioxidant defense and healthy eyes and might prevent/retard/modify AMD. *J Ophthalmol*, 2014;2014:901686.

[4] Cooper, DA, Eldridge, AL, Peters, JC. (1999). Dietary carotenoids and certain cancers, heart disease, and age-related macular degeneration: a review of recent research. *Nutr Rev*, 57(7):201-214.

[5] Chiu, CJ, Milton, RC, Gensler, G, Taylor, A. (2007). Association between dietary glycemic index and age-related macular degeneration in nondiabetic participants in the Age-Related Eye Disease Study. *Am J Clin Nutr*, 86(1):180-8.

[6] McGinness, MB, Karahalios, A, Simpson, JA, Guymer, RH, Robman, LD. (2016). Past physical activity and age-related macular degeneration: the Melbourne Collaborative Cohort Study. *Brit J Ophthalmol*, Oct;100(10):1353-8.

[7] Stanislovaitiene, D, Zaliuniene, D, Krisiukaitis, A, Petrolis, R, Smalinskiene, A. (2017). SCARB1 rs5888 is associated with the risk of age-related macular degeneration susceptibility and an impaired macular area. *Ophthalmic Genet*, May-Jun;38(3):233-237.

[8] Seddon, JM, Willett, WC, Speizer, FE. (1996). A Prospective Study of Cigarette Smoking and Age-Related Macular Degeneration in Women. *JAMA*, Oct 9;276(14):1141-6.

[9] Cederbaum, A. (1989). Role of lipid peroxidation and oxidative stress in alcohol toxicity. *Free Radic Biol Med*, 7:537–5394. Biologically, heavy drinking may cause oxidative damage to the retina leading to the development of AMD.

[10] Obisesan, TO, Hirsch, R, Kosoko, O, Carlson, L, Parrott, M. (1998). Moderate wine consumption is associated with decreased odds of developing age-related macular degeneration in NHANES-1. *J Am Geriatr Soc*, 46:1–7.

[11] Dougherty, BE, Cooley, S L, Davidorf, FH. (2017). Measurement of Perceived Stress in Age-Related Macular Degeneration. *Optom Vis Sci*, Mar;94(3):290-296.

[12] Zhang, QY, Tie, LJ, Wu, SS, Lv, PL, Huang, HW, et al. (2016). Overweight, Obesity, and Risk of Age-Related Macular Degeneration. *Invest Ophthalmol Vis Sci* Mar,57(3):1276-83.

[13] Hyman, L, Schachat, AP, He, Q, Leske, MC. (2000). Hypertension, cardiovascular disease, and age-related macular degeneration. Age-Related Macular Degeneration Risk Factors Study Group. *Arch Ophthalmol*, Mar;118(3):351-8.

[14] Sene A, Khan A, et al. (2013). Impaired cholesterol efflux in senescent macrophages promotes age-related macular degeneration. *Cell Metab*, Apr 2;17(4):549-61.

[15] Feher, J, Kovasc, B, Kovacs, I, Schvoller, M, Papale, A, et al. (2005). Improvement of visual functions and fundus alterations in early age-related macular degeneration treated with a combination of acetyl-L-carnitine, n-3 fatty acids, and coenzyme Q10. *Ophthalmologica*, May-Jun;219(3):154-66.

[16] Ibid. Feher. (2005).

[17] VandenLangenberg, GM, Mares-Perlman, JA, Klein, R, Klein, B, Brady, WE, et al. (1998). Associations between antioxidant and zinc intake and the 5-year incidence of early age-related maculopathy in the Beaver Dam Eye Study. *Am J Epidemiol*, Jul 15;148(2):204-14.

[18] Seddon, JM, George, S, Rosner, B, Rifai, N. (2005). Progression of age-related macular degeneration: prospective assessment of C-reactive protein, interleukin 6, and other cardiovascular biomarkers. *Arch Ophthalmol*, Jun;123(6):774-82.

[19] Seddon, JM, Ajani, UA, Sperduto, RD, Hiller, R, Blair, N, et al. (1994). Dietary carotenoids, vitamins A, C, and E, and advanced age-related

macular degeneration. Eye Disease Case-Control Study Group. *JAMA*, 272(18):1413-1420.

[20] Augood, C, Chakravarthy, U, Young, I, Vioque, J, de Jong, PT, et al. (2008). Oily fish consumption, dietary docosahexaenoic acid and eicosapentaenoic acid intakes, and associations with neovascular age-related macular degeneration. *Am J Clin Nutr*, 88(2): 398–406.

[21] Seddon, JM, Rosner, B, Sperduto, RD, Yannuzzi, L, Haller, JA, et al. (2001). *Dietary fat and risk for advanced age-related macular degeneration.* Arch Ophthalmol. 119(8): 1191–1199.

[22] Sofi, F, Sodi, A, Franco, F, Murro, V, Biagini, D, et al. (2016). Dietary profile of patients with Stargardt's disease and Retinitis Pigmentosa: is there a role for a nutritional approach? *BMC Ophthalmol*, Jan 22;16:13.

[23] Mares-Perlman, JA, Millen, A E, Ficek, TL, Hankinson, SE. (2002). The body of evidence to support a protective role for lutein and zeaxanthin in delaying chronic disease. *J Nutr*, 132(3):518S-524S.

[24] Vives-Bauza, C, Anand, M, Shiraz, AK, Magrane, J, Vollmer-Snarr, H et al. (2008). The age lipid A2E and mitochondrial dysfunction synergistically impair phagocytosis by retinal pigment epithelial cells, *J Bio Chem*, Sep 5;283(36):24770-80.

[25] Ibid. Seddon. (2005).

[26] Ibid. Vives-Bauza. (2008).

[27] Cai, J, Nelson, KC, Wu, M, Sternberg, P, Jones, DP. (2000). Oxidative damage and protection of the RPE. *Prog Ret Eye Res*, 19(2), 205-22.

[28] Boekhoorn, SS, Vingerling, JR, Witteman, JCM, et al. (2007). C-reactive Protein Level and Risk of Aging Macula DisorderThe Rotterdam Study. *Arch Opthalmol*, 125(10):1396-1401.

[29] Shahid, H, Khan, JC, Cipriani, V, Sepp, T, Baljinder, K, et al. (2012). Age-related macular degeneration: the importance of family history as a risk factor. *Br J Ophthalmol*, 96(3):427-431.

[30] Ibid. Shahid. (2012).

[31] Ibid. Shahid. (2012).

[32] Ibid. VandenLangenberg. (1998).

[33] Ibid. VandenLangenberg. (1998).

[34] Buschini, E, Fea, AM, Lavia, CA, Nassasi, M, Pignata, G, et al. (2015). Recent developments in the management of dry age-related macular degeneration. *Clin Ophthalmol*, Apr 1;9:563-74

[35] Hyman, L, Schachat, AP, He, Q, Leske, MC. (2000). Hypertension, cardiovascular disease, and age-related macular degeneration. Age-Related Macular Degeneration Risk Factors Study Group. *Arch Ophthalmol*, Mar;118(3):351-8.

[36] Ibid. Stanislovaitiene. (2017).

[37] Ibid. Seddon. (1996).

[38] Mitta, VP, Chisten, WG, Glynn, RJ, Semba, RD, Ridker, PM, et al. (2013). C-reactive protein and the incidence of macular degeneration: pooled analysis of 5 cohorts. Ophthalmol, Apr;131(4):507-13.

[39] Coral, K, Raman, R, Rathi, S, Rajesh, M, Sulochana, KN, et al. (2005). Plasma homocysteine and total thiol content in patients with exudative age-related macular degeneration. *Eye (Lond)*, Feb;20(2):203-7

[40] Huang, P, Wang, F, Sah, BK, Jiang, J, Ni, Z, et al. (2015). Homocysteine and the risk of age-related macular degeneration: a systematic review and meta-analysis. *Sci Rep*, Jul 21;5:10585.

[41] Feskanich, D, Cho, E, Schaumberg, DA, Colditz, GA, Hankinson, SE. (2008). Menopausal and Reproductive Factors and Risk of Age-Related Macular Degeneration. *Arch Ophthalmol*, Apr;126(4):519-24

[42] Mares-Perlman JA, Millen AE, Ficek TL, Hankinson SE. The body of evidence to support a protective role for lutein and zeaxanthin in delaying chronic disease. Overview. *J Nutr*, 2002;132(3):518S-524S.

[43] American Macular Degeneration Foundation. Medication Cautions in Macular Degeneration. Retrieved Sep 21 2017 from https://www.macular.org/medications-use-caution.

[44] Wu, J, Uchino, M, Sastry, SM, Schumberg, D. (2014). Age-Related Macular Degeneration and the Incidence of Cardiovascular Disease: A Systematic Review and Meta-Analysis. *PLoS One*, 2014; 9(3): e89600.

[45] Bleich, S, Roedl, J, Von Ahsen, N, Schlotzer-Schrehardt, U, Reulbach, U, et al. (2004). Elevated homocysteine levels in aqueous humor of patients with pseudoexfoliation glaucoma. *Am J Ophthalmol,* Jul;138(1):162-4.

[46] Parisi, V, Tedeschi, M, Gallianaro, G, Varano, M, Saviano, S, et al. (2008). Carotenoids and antioxidants in age-related maculopathy: multifocal electroretinogram modifications after 1 year. *Ophthalmology,* Feb;115(2):324-333.e2.

[47] Piermarocchi, S, Saviano, S, Parisi, V, Tedeschi, M, Panozzo, G, et al. (2012). Carotenoids in Age-related Maculopathy Italian Study (CARMIS): two-year results of a randomized study. *Eur J Ophthalmol,* Mar-Apr;22(2):216-25.

[48]National Eye Institute. (2013). NIH Study provides clarity on supplements for protection against blinding eye disease. Retrieved June 10 2017 from https://nei.nih.gov/news/pressreleases/050513.

[49] AREDS, AREDS2: (2001, 2006, 2013) Antioxidants & Macular Degeneration. Retrieved on Oct 15 2017 from http://www.naturaleyecare.com/study.asp?s_num=105.

[50] Snellen, EL, Verbeek, AL, Van Den Hoogen, GW, Crysberg, JR, Hoyng, CB. (2002). Neovascular age-related macular degeneration and its relationship to antioxidant intake. *Acta Ophthalmol Scand,* Aug;80(4):368-71.

[51] Richer, S, Stiles, W, Statkute, L, Pulido, J, Frankowski, J, et al. (2004). Double-masked, placebo-controlled, randomized trial of lutein and antioxidant supplementation in the intervention of atrophic age-related macular degeneration: the Veterans LAST study (Lutein Antioxidant Supplementation Trial). *Optometry,* Apr;75(4):216-30.

[52] Souied, EH, Delcourt, C, Querques, G, Bassols, A, Merle, B, et al. (2013). Oral docosahexaenoic acid in the prevention of exudative age-related macular degeneration: The Nutritional AMD Treatment 2 Study. *Ophthalmology,* Aug;120(8):1619-31.

[53] Landrum, JT, Bone, RA, Joa, H, Kilburn, MD, Moore, LL, et al. (1997). A one year study of the macular pigment: the effect of 140 days of a lutein supplement. *Exp Eye Res,* Jul;65(1):57-62.

54 Bernstein, PS, Zhao, DY, Wintch, SW, Ermakov, IV, McClane, RW, et al. (2002). Resonance Raman measurement of macular carotenoids in normal subjects and in age-related macular degeneration patients. *Ophthalmology*, Oct;109(10):1780-7.

55 Seddon, JM, Ajani, UA, Sperduto, RD, Hiller, R, Blair, N, et al, (1994). Dietary carotenoid, vitamins A, C, E, and advanced age-related macular degeneration. *JAMA*, Nov 9;272(18):1413-20.

56 Landrum, JT, Bone, RA, Kilburn, MD. (1997). The Macular Pigment: A Possible Role in Protection from Age-Related Macular Degeneration. *Adv Pharmacol*, 38:537-56.

57 Ibid. Landrum. (1997).

58 Ibid. Landrum. (1997).

59Semba, RD, Dagnelie, G. (2003). Are lutein and zeaxanthin conditionally essential nutrients for eye health? *Med Hypotheses*, Oct;61(4):465-72.

60Krinsky, NI, Landrum, JT, Bone, RA. (2003). Biologic mechanisms of the protective role of lutein and zeaxanthin in the eye. *Annu Rev Nutr*, 23:171-201.

61Koushan, K, Rusovici, R, Li, W, Ferguson, LR, Chalam, KV. (2013). The Role of Lutein in Eye-Related Disease. *Nutrients*, May; 5(5): 1823–1839.

62 Kijlstra, A, Tian, Y, Kelly, ER, Berendschot, TT. (2012). Lutein: more than just a filter for blue light. *Prog Ret Eye Res*, Jul;31(4):303-15.

63 Chung HY, Rasmussen HM, Johnson EJ. (2004) Lutein bioavailability is higher from lutein-enriched eggs than from supplements and spinach in men. *J Nutr*, Aug;134(8):1887-93.

64Estevez-Santiago, R, Olmedilla-Alonso, B, Beltran-de-Miguel, B, Cuadrado-Vives, C. (2016). Lutein and zeaxanthin supplied by red/orange foods and fruits are more closely associated with macular pigment optical density than those from green vegetables in Spanish subjects. *Nutr Res*, Nov;36(11):1210-1221.

65Li, B, Ahmed, F, Bernstein, PS. (2010). Studies on the singlet oxygen scavenging mechanism of human macular pigment. *Arch Biochem Biophys*, Dec 1;504 (1): 56–60.

[66] Bone, RA, Landrum, JT, Cao, Y, Howard, AN, Alvarez-Calderon, F. (2007). Macular pigment response to a supplement containing meso-zeaxanthin, lutein and zeaxanthin. *Nutr Metab (Lond),* Pub. online May 11.

[67] Ma, L, Liu, R, Du, JH, Liu, T, Wu, SS. (2016). Lutein, Zeaxanthin and Meso-zeaxanthin Supplementation Associated with Macular Pigment Optical Density. *Nutrients,* Jul 12;8(7):E426.

[68] Ibid. Ma. (2016).

[69] Delcourt, C, Carriere, I, Delage, M, Barberger-Gateau, P, Schalch, W. (2006). Plasma Lutein and Zeaxanthin and Other Carotenoids as Modifiable Risk Factors for Age-Related Maculopathy and Cataract: The POLA Study. *Inves Ophthal Vis Sci,* Jun:47:2329-35.

[70] Herman, JP, Kleiner-Goudey, SJ, Davis, RL. (2017). Dietary Supplements Improving Macular and Visual Function. *Adv Ophthal Vis Syst,* Dec;6(1):00166.

[71]Richer, SP, Stiles, W, Graham-Hoffman, K, Levin, M, Ruskin, D, et al. (2011). Randomized, double-blind, placebo-controlled study of zeaxanthin and visual function in patients with atrophic age-related macular degeneration: the Zeaxanthin and Visual Function Study (ZVF) FDA IND #78, 973. *Optometry,* Nov;82(11):667-680.e6.

[72]Ibid. Richer. (2011).

[73] Ibid.Delcourt. (2006).

[74] Ibid. Richer. (2011).

[75] Stringham, JM, O'Brien, KJ, Stringham, NT. (2016). Macular carotenoid supplementation improves disability glare performance and dynamics of photostress recovery. *Eye Vis (Lond),* Nov11;3:30.

[76] Omega-3 fatty acid, Wikipedia, Retrieved Nov 18 2017 from https://en.wikipedia.org/wiki/Omega-3_fatty_acid

[77] Anderson, MB, Ma, DWL. (2009). Are all n-3 polyunsaturated fatty acids created equal? *Lip Health Dis,* Aug 10;8:33.

[78] Ibid. Delcourt. (2006).

[79] Ibid. Merle. (2001).

[80] Ibid. Smith. (2000).

[81] Ibid. Seddon. (2001).

[82] Ibid. SanGiovanni. (2005).

[83] Ibid. Cho. (2001).

[84] Delcourt C, Carriere I, Cristol, JP, Lacroux, A, Gerber, M. (2007). Dietary fat and the risk of age-related maculopathy: the POLANUT Study. *Euro J Clin Nutr*, Nov;61(11):1341-4.

[85] Ibid. Chong. (2008).

[86] Chong, EW, Robman, LD, Simpson, JA, Hodge, AM, Aung, KZ, et al. (2009). Fat consumption and its association with age-related macular degeneration. *Arch Ophthalmol,* May;127(5):674-80.

[87]Connor, WE, Neuringer, M, Reisbick, S. (1992). Essential fatty acids: The importance of n-2 fatty acids in the retina and the brain. *Nutr Rev,* Apr;50(4(Pt2)):21-29.

[88] Chong, EW, Kris, AJ, Wong, TY, Simpson, JA, Guymer, RH. (2008). Dietary omega-3 fatty acid and fish intake in the primary prevention of age-related macular degeneration: a systematic review and meta-analysis. *Arch Opthalmol,* Jun;126(6):826-33.

[89]SanGiovanni, JP, Agron, E, Meleth, AD, Reed, GF, Sperduto, RD, et al. (2009). Omega-3 Long-chain polyunsaturated fatty acid intake and 12-y incidence of neovascular age-related macular degeneration and central geographic atrophy: AREDS report 30, a prospective cohort study from the Age-Related Eye Disease Study. *Am J C Nutr,* Dec;90(6):1601-7.

[90]Christen, WG, Schaumberg, DA, Glynn, RJ, Buring, JE. (2011). Dietary omega-3 fatty acid and fish intake and incident age-related macular degeneration in women. *Arch Ophthalmol,* Jul;129(7):921-9.

[91]Mukherjee, PK, Marcheselli, VL, Serhan, CN, Bazan, NG. (2004). Neuroprotectin D1: a docosahexaenoic acid-derived docosatriene protects human retinal pigment epithelial cells from oxidative stress. *Proc Natl Acad Sci USA,* Jun 1;101(22):8491-6.

[92] Ibid. Querques. (2011).

93 Calder, PC. (2015). Marine omega-3 fatty acids and inflammatory processes: Effects, mechanisms and clinical relevance. *Biochem Biophys Acta,* Apr;1851(4):469-84.

94Chen, W, Esselman, WJ, Jump, DB, Busik, JV. (2005). Anti-inflammatory effect of docosahexaenoic acid on cytokine-induced adhesion molecule expression in human retinal vascular endothelial cells. *Invest Ophthalmol Vis Sci,* Nov;46(11):4342-7.

95 Ibid. Querques. (2011).

96 Orr, SK, Palumbo, S, Bosetti, F, Mount, HT, Kang, JX, et al. (2013). Unesterified docosahexaenoic acid is protective in neuroinflammation. *J Neurochem,* Nov;127(3):378–393.

97 Ibid. Querques. (2011).

98SanGiovanni, JP, Chew, EY. (2005). The role of omega-3 long-chain polyunsaturated fatty acids in health and disease of the retina. *Prog Retin Eye Res,* 2005;24(1): 87–138.

99 Yanai, R, Mulki, L, Hasegawa, E, Takeuchi, K Sweigad, H, et al. (2014). Cytochrome P450-generated metabolites derived from omega-3 fatty acids attenuate neovascularization. *Proc Natl Acad Sci U S A,* Jul 1;111(26):9603-8.

100Bazan, NG. (2006). Cell survival matters: docosahexaenoic acid signaling, neuroprotection and photoreceptors. *Trends Neurosci,* May;29(5):263-71.

101 Lacon, A, Frazzi, R, Latruffe, N. (2016). Anti-Oxidant, Anti-Inflammatory and Anti-angiogenic Properties of Resveratrol in Ocular Disease. *Molecules.* Mar 2;21(3):304.

102 Kang, JH, Choung, SY. (2016). Protective effects of resveratrol and its analogs on age-related macular degeneration in vitro. *Arch Pharm Res.* Dec;30(12):1703-1715.

103 Abu-Amero, KK, Kondkar, AA, Chalam, KV. (2016). Resveratrol and Ophthalmic diseases. *Nutrients,* Apr 5;8(4):200.

104 Ibid. Wang. (2014).

[105] Wang, S, Wang, Z, Yang, S, Yin, T, Zhang, Y. (2017). Tissue Distribution of trans-Resveratrol and Its Metabolites after Oral Administration in Human Eyes, *J Ophthalmol*, 4052094, 12 pp.

[106] Ibid. Niesen. (2013).

[107] Bola, C, Bartlett, H, Eperjesi, F. (2014). Resveratrol and the eye: activity and molecular mechanisms. *Graefes Arch Clin Exp Ophthalmol*, May;252(5);699-713.

[108] Ibid. Bola. (2014).

[109] Ibid. Abu-Amero. (2016).

[110] Ibid. Niesen. (2013).

[111] Ibid. Wang. (2017).

[112] Vitseva, O, Varghese, S, Chakrabarti, S, Folts, JD, Freedman, JE. (2005). Grape seed and skin extracts inhibit platelet function and release of reactive oxygen intermediates. *J Cardiovasc Pharmacol*, Oct;46(4):445-51.

[113] Balu, M, Sangeetha, P, Murali, G, Panneerselvam, C. (2005). Age-related oxidative protein damages in central nervous system of rats: modulatory role of grape seed extract. *Int J Dev Neurosci*, Oct;23(6):501-7.

[114] Marangoni, D, Falsini, B, Piccardi, M, Ambrosio, L, Minnella, AM, et al. (2013). Functional effect of Saffron supplementation and risk genotypes in early age-related macular degeneration: a preliminary report. *J Transl Med*, Sep;11:228.

[115] Alavizadeh, SH, Hosseinzadeh, H. (2014). Bioactivity assessment and toxicity of crocin: a comprehensive review. *Food Chem Toxicol*, Feb;64:65-80.

[116] Broadhead, GK, Grigg, JR, Chang, AA, McCluskey, P. (2015). Dietary modification and supplementation for the treatment of age-related macular degeneration. *Nutr Rev*, Jul;73(7):448-62.

[117] Broadhead, GK, Chang, A, Grigg, J, McCluskey, P. (2016). Efficacy and Safety of Saffron Supplementation: Current Clinical Findings. *Cril Rev Food Sci Nutr*, Dec 9;56(16):2767-76.

[118] Corso, L, Cavallero, A, Baroni, D, Garbati, P, Prestipino, G, et al. (2016). Saffron reduces ATP-induced retinal cytotoxicity by targeting P2X7 receptors. *Purinergic Signal*, Mar;12(1):161-74.

[119] Bisti, S, Maccarone, R, Falsini, B. (2014). Saffron and retina: neuroprotection and pharmacokinetics. *Vis Neurosci*, Sep;31(4-5):355-61.

[120] Lashay, A, Sadough, G, Ashrafi, E, Lasay, M, Movassat, M, et al. (2016). Short-term Outcomes of Saffron Supplementation in Patients with Age-related Macular Degeneration: A Double-blind, Placebo-controlled, Randomized Trial. *Med Hypothesis Discov Innov Ophthalmol.* Spring;5(1)32-38.

[121] Falsini, B, Piccardi, M, Minnella, A, Savastano, C, Capoluongo, E, et al. (2010). Influence of saffron supplementation on retinal flicker sensitivity in early age-related macular degeneration, *Invest Ophthalmol Vis Sci*, Dec;51(12):6118-24.

[122] Marangoni, D, Falsini, B, Piccardi, M, Ambrosio, L, Minnella, AM. (2013). Functional effect of saffron supplementation and risk genotypes in early age-related macular degeneration: a preliminary report, *J Transl Med*, Sep 25;11:228.

[123]Cangemi, R, Angelico, F, Loffredo, L, Del Ben, M, Pignatelli, P, et al. (2007). Oxidative stress-mediated arterial dysfunction in patients with metabolic syndrome: Effect of ascorbic acid. *Free Radic Biol Med*, Sep 1;43(5):853-9.

[124] Chew, EY, Clemons, TE, Agron, E, Sperduto, RE, Sangiovanni, JP, et al. (2013). Long-term effects of vitamins C and E, β-carotene, and zinc on age-related macular degeneration: AREDS report no. 35. *Opthalmology*, Aug;120(8):1604-11.

[125] Du, J, Cullen, JJ, Buettner, GR. (2012). Ascorbic acid: chemistry, biology and the treatment of cancer. *Biochem Biophys Acta*, Dec;1826(2):443-57.

[126] Ibid. AREDS Research Group. (2001).

[127] Ibid. Cho. (2004).

[128]Tanumihardjo, SK, Li, J, Dosti, MP. (2005). Lutein absorption is facilitated with co-supplementation of ascorbic acid in young adults. *J Am Dietetic Assoc,* 105:114-18.

[129] AREDS, AREDS2: (2001, 2006, 2013) Antioxidants & Macular Degeneration. Retrieved on Oct 15 2017 from http://www.naturaleyecare.com/study.asp?s_num=105.

[130] Wikipedia. Vitamin D. Retrieved Nov 2 2017 from https://en.wikipedia.org/wiki/Vitamin_D.

[131] Dietobio. Vitamin D. Retrieved Nov 2 2017 from http://www.dietobio.com/vegetarisme/en/vit_d.html

[132] Millen, AE, Meyers, KJ, Liu, Z, Engelman, CD, Wallace, RB, et al. (2015). Association between vitamin D status and age-related macular degeneration by genetic risk. *JAMA Ophthalmol,* Oct: 133(10: 1171-79.

[133] Vitamin D linked to lower macular degeneration risk. (2016). Naturaleyecare. Retrieved Nov 2 2017 from http://www.naturaleyecare.com/blog/vitamin-d-linked-to-lower-macular-degeneration-risk.

[134]Mutlu, U, Ikram, MA, Hofman, A, de Jong, PT, Uitterlinden, AG, et al. (2016). Vitamin D and retinal microvascular damage: The Rotterdam Study. *Medicine (Baltimore),* Dec; 95(49): e5477.

[135] Belda, JI, Roma, J, Vielela, C, Puertas, FJ, Diaz-Llopis, M, Bosch-Morell, F, et al. (1999). Serum vitamin E levels negatively correlate with severity of age-related macular degeneration, *Mech Ageing Dev,* Mar 1;107(2):159-64.

[136] Chew, EY, Clemons, TE, Agron, E, Sperduto, RD, Sangiovanni, JP. (2013). Long-term effects of vitamins C and E, beta carotene, and zinc on age-related macular degeneration: AREDS report no. 35. *Ophthalmology,* Aug;120(8):1604-11.

[137] Qing, J. (2014). Natural forms of vitamin E: metabolism, antioxidant and anti-inflammatory activities and the role in disease prevention and therapy. *Free Radic Biol Med,* Jul;72:76–90.

[138] Lewis, EE, Meydani, SN, Wu, D. (2019). Regulatory role of vitamin E in the immune system and inflammation. *IUBMB Life.* Apr;71(4):487-494.

[139] Piermarocchi, S, Saviano, S, Parisi, V, Tedeschi, M, Panozzo, G, et al. (2012). Carotenoids in Age-related Maculopathy Italian Study (CARMIS): two-year results of a randomized study. *Eur J Ophthalmol*, Mar-Apr;22(2):216-25.

[140] Otsuka, T, Shimazawa, M, Nakanishi, T, Ohno, Y, Inoue, Y, et al. (2013). Protective effects of a dietary carotenoid, astaxanthin, against light-induced retinal damage. *J Pharmacol Sci*, 123(3):209-18.

[141] Ibid. Otsuka. (2013).

[142] Inoue, Y, Shimazawa, M, Nagano, R, Kuse, Y, Takahashi, K. (2017), Astaxanthin analogs, adonixanthin and lycopene, activate Nrf2 to prevent light-induced photoreceptor degeneration. *J Pharmacol Sci*, Jul;134(3):147-157.

[143] Ibid. He. (2011).

[144] Yigit, M, Gunes, A, Uguz, C, Yalcin, TO, Tok, L, et al. (2019). Effects of astaxanthin on antioxidant parameters in ARPE-19 cells on oxidative stress model. *Int J Ophthalmol.* Jun 18;12(6):930-935.

[145] Kidd, P. (2011). Astaxanthin, cell membrane nutrient with diverse clinical benefits and anti-aging potential. *Alt Med Rev*, Dec;16(4):355-64).

[146] De Jesus Raposo, MF, de Morais, AM, de Morais, RM. (2015). Carotenoids from Marine Microalgae: A Valuable Natural Source for the Prevention of Chronic Diseases. *Mar Drugs*, Aug;13(8):5128-5155.

[147] Sawaki, K, Yoshigi, H, Aoki, K, Koikawa, N, Zaumane, A, et al. (2002). Sports performance benefits from taking natural astaxanthin characterized by visual acuity and muscle fatigue improvement in humans. *J Clin Ther Med*, 18(9)1085-1100.

[148] Ibid. Kidd. (2011).

[149] Maher, TJ. (2000). Astaxanthin, Continuing Ed Module., New Hope Institute of Healing.

[150]Goto, S, Kogure, K, Abe, K, Kimata, Y, Kitahama, K, et al. (2001). Efficient radical trapping at the surface and inside the phospholipid membrane is responsible for highly potent antiperoxidative activity of the carotenoid astaxanthin. *Biochimica Biophysica Acta*, 1512:251-8.

[151]BetaForce. Astaxanthin: The Most Powerful Natural Antioxidant Ever Discovered. Retrieved Apr 2 2018 from http://www.beta-glucan-info.com/astaxanthin.htm.

[152]Chiro.org. Antioxidants: Relative Singlet Oxygen Quenching Rates. Retrieved Apr 16 2018 from http://www.chiro.org/nutrition/FULL/ Antioxidants_Relative_Singlet_Oxygen_Quenching_Rates.html.

[153]Lee, SJ, Bai, SK, et al, (2003), Astaxanthin inhibits nitric oxide production and inflammatory gene expression by suppressing I(kappa)B kinase-dependent NF-kappaB activation. *Mol Cells*, Aug 31;16(1):97-105.

[154] Astaxanthin (2002-2006) Reduces Eye Fatigue. Retrieved Nov 10 2017 from http://www.naturaleyecare.com/study.asp?s_num=272.

[155]Nagaki, Y, Hayasaka, S, Yamad, a T, Hayasaka, Y, Sanada, M, et al. (2002). Effects of astaxanthin on accommodation, critical flicker fusions, and pattern evoked potential in visual display terminal workers. *J Trad Med*, 19(5):170-173.

[156] Ibid. Nagaki. (2002).

[157]Nakamura, A, Isobe, R, Otaka, Y, Abematsu, Y, Nakata, D, et al. (2004). Changes in Visual Function Following Peroral Astaxanthin. *Japan J Cli Opthal*, 58(6):1051-1054.

[158]Takahashi, N, Kajita, M. (2005). Effects of astaxanthin on accommodative recovery. *J Clin Therap Med*, 21(4):431-436.

[159] Ogami, SK. (2010). Effect of astaxanthin on accommodation and asthenopia Efficacy identification study in healthy volunteers. *J Clin Ther Med*, 21(5):543-556.

[160]Iwasaki, T, Tawara, A. (2006). Effects of Astaxanthin on Eyestrain Induced by Accommodative Dysfunction. *J Eye (Atarashii Ganka)*, Jun;23(6):829-834.

[161]Camire ME. (2000). *Herbs, Botanicals and Teas*. Bilberries and blueberries as functional foods and nutraceuticals; pp. 289–319. Lancaster, PA: Technomic Publishing Company.

[162]Chu, WK, Cheung, SCM, Lau, RAW, Benzie, IFF. (2011). Chapter 4 Bilberry (Vaccinium myrtillus L.). *Herbal Medicine: Biomecular and Clinical Aspects. 2nd ed.* Boca Raton, FL: CRC Press/Taylor & Francis.

[163]Kemper, KJ. (1965). Bilberry (Vaccinium myrtillus). *Ann Ottalmol Clin Ocul*,1965;91:371-86.

[164]Upton, R, editor. (2001). Bilberry Fruit Vaccinium myrtillus L. Standards of Analysis, Quality Control, and Therapeutics. *American Herbal Pharmacopoeia and Therapeutic Compendium.* Santa Cruz, CA.

[165] Osada, H, Okamoto, T, Kawashima, H, Toda, E, Miyake, S, et al. (2017). Neuroprotective effect of bilberry extract in a murine model of photo-stressed retina. *PLoS One*, Jun 1;12(6):e0178627.

[166]Wang, Y, Zhao, L, Lu, F, Yang, X, Deng, Q, et al. (2015). Retinoprotective Effects of Bilberry Anthocyanins via Antioxidant, Anti-Inflammatory, and Anti-Apoptotic Mechanisms in a Visible Light-Induced Retinal Degeneration Model in Pigmented Rabbits. *Molecules,* Dec 14;20(12):22395-410.

[167]Zafra-Stone, S, Yasmin, T, Bagchi, M, Chatterjee, A, Vinson, JA, et al. (2007). Berry anthocyanins as novel antioxidants in human health and disease prevention. *Mol Nutr Food Res*, Jun;51(6):675-83.

[168] Mastantuono, T, Starita, N, Sapio, D, D'Avanzo, SA, Di Maro, M, et al. (2016). The Effects of Vaccinium myrtillus Extract on Hamster Pial Microcirculation during Hypoperfusion-Reperfusion Injury. *PLoS One,* Apr 12;11(4):e0150659.

[169]Cohen-Boulakia, F, Valensi, PE, Boulahdour, H, Lestrade, R, Dufour-Lamarinie, JF, et al. (2000). In vivo sequential study of skeletal muscle capillary permeability in diabetic rats: effect of anthocyanosides. *Metabolism,* Jul;49(7):880-5.

[170] Muth, ER, Laurent, JM, Jasper, P. (2000). The effect of bilberry nutritional supplementation on night visual acuity and contrast sensitivity. *Altern Med Rev,* Apr;5(2):164-73.

[171] Matsunaga, N, Imai, S, Inokuchi, Y, Shimazawa, M, Yokota, S, et al. (2009). Bilberry and its main constituents have neuroprotective effects

against retinal neuronal damage in vitro and in vivo. *Mol Nutr Food Res*, Jul;53(7):869-77.

[172] Yao, Y, Vieria, A. (2007). Protective activities of Vaccinium antioxidants with potential relevance to mitochondrial dysfunction and neurotoxicity. *Neurotoxicology,* 28 93–100.

[173] Colantuoini, A, Bertuglia, S, Magistretti, MJ, Donato, L. (1991). Effects of Vaccinium Myrtillus anthocyanosides on arterial vasomotion. *Arzneimittelforschung*, Sep;41(9):905-9.

[174]Zhu, Y, Xia, M, Yang, Y, Liu, F, Li, Z, et al. (2011). Purified anthocyanin supplementation improves endothelial function via NO-cGMP activation in hypercholesterolemic individuals. *Clin Chem,* Nov;57(11):1524-33.

[175] Yamaura, K, Simada, M, Ueno, K. (2011). Anthocyanins from bilberry (Vaccinium myrtillus L.) alleviate pruritus in a mouse model of chronic allergic contact dermatitis. *Pharmacogosy Res*, Jul;3(3):173-7.

[176] Ibid. Matsunaga. (2009).

[177]Mazza, G, Kay, CD, Correll, T, Holub, BJ. (2002). Absorption of anthocyanins from blueberries and serum antioxidant status in human subjects. *J Agric Food Chem*, 50:7731–7.

[178] Saberi-Karimian, M, Katsiki, M, Caraglia, M, Boccellino, M, Majeed, M, et al. (2017). Vascular endothelial growth factor: An important molecular target of curcumin. *Crit Rev Food Sci Nutr*, Aug 30:1-14.

[179]Woo, JM, Shin, DY, Lee, SJ, Joe, Y, Zheng, M, et al. (2012). Curcumin protects retinal pigment epithelial cells against oxidative stress via induction of heme oxygenase-1 expression and reduction of reactive oxygen. *Mol Vis*, 18: 901–908.

[180] Park, SI, Lee, EH, Kim, SR, Jang, YP. (2017). Anti-apoptotic effects of Curcuma longa L. extract and its curcuminoids against blue light-induced cytotoxicity in A2E-laden human retinal pigment epithelial cells. *J Pharm Pharacol*, Mar;69(3):334-340.

[181] Zhu, W, Wu, Y, Meng, YF, Wang, JY, Xu, M, et al. (2015). Effect of curcumin on aging retinal pigment epithelial cells. *Drug Des Devel Ther*, Sep 25;9:5337-44.

[182]Calabrese, V, Bates, TE, Mancuso, C, Cornelius, C, Ventimiglia, B, et al. (2008). Curcumin and the cellular stress response in free radical-related diseases. *Mol Nutr Food Res,* Sep;52(9):1062-73.

[183]Mashayekh, A, Pham, DL, Yousem, DM, Dizon, M, Barker, PB, et al. (2011). Effects of Ginkgo biloba on cerebral blood flow assessed by quantitative MR perfusion imaging: a pilot study. *Neuroradiology,* Mar;53(3):185-191.

[184] Principles of herbal pharmacology. (2013). In Bone, K. and Mills, S. (Eds.), *Principles and Practice of Phytotherapy: Modern Herbal Medicine.* St. Louis, Mo: Elsevier Sanders.

[185]Fies, P, Dienel, A. (2002). Ginkgo extract in impaired vision--treatment with special extract EGb 761 of impaired vision due to dry senile macular degeneration. *Wien Med Wochenschr,*2002;152(15-16):423-6.

[186]Lebuisson, DA, Leroy, L, Rigal, G. (1986). Treatment of senile macular degeneration with Ginkgo biloba extract. A preliminary double-blind drug vs. placebo study. *Presse Med,* Sep 25;15(31):1556-8.

[187] Diamond, BJ, Shiflett, SC, Feiwel, N, Matheis, RJ, Noskin, O, et al. (2000). Ginkgo biloba extract: mechanisms and clinical indications. *Arch Phys Med Rehabil,* May;81(5):668-78.

[188] Oh, JH, Oh, J, Togloom, A, Kim, SW, Huh, K. (2013). Effects of Ginkgo biloba Extract on Cultured Human Retinal Pigment Epithelial Cells under Chemical Hypoxia. *Curr Eye Res,* Oct;38(10): 1072–1082.

[189] Droy-Lefaix, MT, Cluzel, J, Menerath, JM, Bonhomme, B, Doly, M. (1995). Antioxidant effect of a Ginkgo biloba extract (EGb 761) on the retina. *Antint J Tissue React,*1995;17(3):93-100.

[190] Ayalaxomayajula, SP, Kompella, UB. (2002). Induction of vascular endothelial growth factor by 4-hydroxynonenal and its prevention by glutathione precursors in retinal pigment epithelial cells. *Eur J Pharmacol,* Aug 9;449(3):213-20.

[191] Qin, L, Mroczkowska, SA, Ekart, A, Patel, SR, Gibson, JM, et al. (2014). Patients with early age-related macular degeneration exhibit signs of macro- and micro-vascular disease and abnormal blood glutathione levels. *Graefes Arch Clin Exp Ophthalmol,* Jan;252(1):23-30.

[192] Sternberg, P, Davidson, PC, Jones, DP, Hagen, TM, Reed, RL, et al. (1993). Protection of retinal pigment epithelium from oxidative injury by glutathione and precursors. *Invest Ophthalmol Vis Sci, Dec*;34(13):3661-8.

[193] Hall, AG. (1999). The role of glutathione in the regulation of apoptosis. *Eur J Clin Invest*, Mar; 29(3):238-45.

[194] Birdsall, TC. (1998). Therapeutic applications of taurine. *Altern Med Rev*, Apr;3(2):128-36.

[195] Shpak, NI, Naritsyna, NI, Konovalova, NV. (1989). Taufon and emoksipin in the combined treatment of sclerotic macular dystrophies. *Oftalmol Zh*, (8):463-5.

[196] Lombardini, JB. (1991). Taurine: retinal function. *Brain Res Brain Res Rev*, May-Aug;16(2):151-69.

[197] Ibid. Birdsall. (1998).

[198] Ibid. Shpak. (1989).

[199] Ibid. Birdsall. (1998).

[200] Froger, N, Cadetti, L, Lorach, H, Martins, J, Bemelmans, AP, et al. (2012). Taurine provides neuroprotection against retinal ganglion cell degeneration. *PLoS One*,2012;7(10):342017.

[201] Imaki, H, Moretz, R, Wisniewski, H, Neuringer, M, Sturman, J. (1987). Retinal degeneration in 3-month-old rhesus monkey infants fed a taurine-free human infant formula. *J Neurosci Res*, 18(4):602-14.

[202] Lombardini, JB. (1991). Taurine: retinal function. *Brain Res Brain Res Rev*, May-Aug;16(2):151-69.

[203] Petrosian, AM, Haroutounian, JE. (1998). The role of taurine in osmotic, mechanical, and chemical protection of the retinal rod outer segments, *Adv Exp Med Biol*, 442:407-13.

[204] Dhuique-Mayer, C, Servent, A, Descalzo, A, Mouquet-Rivier, C, Amiot, MJ, et al. (2016). Culinary practices mimicking a polysaccharide-rich recipe enhance the bioaccessibility of fat-soluble micronutrients. *Food Chem*, Nov 1;210:182-8.

[205] Linus Pauling Institute. (2016). Carotenoids: α-Carotene, β-Carotene, β-Cryptoxanthin, Lycopene, Lutein, and Zeaxanthin. Retrieved Jul 18

2017 from http://lpi.oregonstate.edu/mic/dietary-factors/phytochemicals/carotenoids.

[206] Mares-Perlman, JA, Brady, WE, Klein, R, Klein, BE, Bowen, P, et al. (1995). Serum antioxidants and age-related macular degeneration in a population-based case-control study. *Arch Ophthalmol*, Dec;113(12):1518

[207] Di Mascio, P, Kaiser, S, Sies, H. (1989). Lycopene as the most efficient biological carotenoid singlet oxygen quencher. *Arch Biochem Biophys*, Nov 1;274(2):532-8.

[208] Erdman, JW, Ford, NA, Lindshield, BL. (2009). Are the health attributes of lycopene related to its antioxidant function? *Arch Biochem Biophys*, Mar 15;483(2):229-35.

[209]Zhao, B, Ren, B, Guo, R, Zhang, W, Ma, S, et al, (2017). Supplementation of lycopene attenuates oxidative stress induced neuroinflammation and cognitive impairment via Nrf2/NF-κB transcriptional pathway. *Food Chem Toxicol*, Nov;109(Pt 1):505-516.

[210] Stefanova, NA, Zhdankina, AA, Fursova, AZ, Kolosova, NG. (2013). Potential of melatonin for prevention of age-related macular degeneration: experimental study. *Adv Gerontol*, 26(1):122-9.

[211] Yi, C, Pan, X, Yan, H, Guo, M, Pierpaoli, W. (2005). Effects of melatonin in age-related macular degeneration. *Ann N Y Acad Sci*, Dec;1057:384-92.

[212] Dieguez, HH, Gonzalez, FMF, Aranda, ML, Calanni, JS, Keller, SMI, et al. (2020). Melatonin protects the retina from experimental nonexudative age-related macular degeneration in mice. *J Pineal Res.* Mar 4;312643.

[213] Mehrzadi, S, Hemati, K, Reiter, RJ, Housseinzadeh, A. (2020). Mitochondrial dysfunction in age-related macular degeneration: melatonin as a potential treatment. Expert Opin Ther Targets. Apr;24(4):359-378.

[214] Zhuang, P, Shen, Y, Lin, BQ, Zhang, WY, Chiou, GC. (2011). Effect of quercetin on formation of choroidal neovascularization (CNV) in age-related macular degeneration (AMD). *Eye Sci*, Mar;26(1):23-9.

[215] Ibid. Zhuang. (2011).

[216]Mitchell, AE, Hong, YJ, Barrett, DM, Bryant, DE, Denison, RF, et al. (2007). Ten-Year Comparison of the Influence of Organic and

Conventional Crop Management Practices on the Content of Flavonoids in Tomatoes. *J Agric Food Chem*, Jul 25;55(15):6154-9.

[217] Quercitin. RxList. Retrieved Sep 18 2017 from https://www.rxlist.com/quercetin-page3/supplements.htm.

[218] Samuel, T, Fadlalla, K, Turner, T, Yehualaeshet, TE. (2010). The flavonoid quercetin transiently inhibits the activity of taxol and nocodazole through interference with the cell cycle. *Nutr Cancer*, (8):1025-35.

[219] Zinc. Wikipedia. Retrieved Nov 2 2017 from https://en.wikipedia.org/wiki/Zinc

[220] Age-Related Eye Disease Study Research Group. (2001). A randomized, placebo-controlled, clinical trial of high-dose supplementation with vitamins C and E, beta carotene, and zinc for age-related macular degeneration and vision loss: AREDS report no. 8. Arch Ophthalmol, 119(10):1417–1436.

[221] AREDS, AREDS2: (2001, 2006, 2013) Antioxidants & Macular Degeneration. Retrieved on Oct 15 2017 from http://www.naturaleyecare.com/study.asp?s_num=105.

[222] Lee, HS, Jun, JH, Jung, EH, Koo, BA, Kim, YS. (2014). Epigalloccatechin-3-gallate inhibits ocular neovascularization and vascular permeability in human retinal pigment epithelial and human retinal microvascular endothelial cells via suppression of MMP-9 and VEGF activation. *Molecules*, Aug 13;19(8):12150-72.

[223] Cia, D, Vergnaud-Gauduchon, J, Jacquemot, N, Doly, M. (2014). Epigallocatechin gallate (EGCG) prevents H2O2-induced oxidative stress in primary rat retinal pigment epithelial cells. *Curr Eye Res*, Sep;39(9):944-52.

[224] Li, CP, Yao, J, Tao, ZF, Li, XM, Jiang, Q, Yan, B. (2013). Epigallocatechin-gallate (EGCG) regulates autophagy in human retinal pigment epithelial cells: a potential role for reducing UVB light-induced retinal damage. *Biochem Biophys Res Commun*, Sep 6;438(4):739-45.

[225] Chu, KO, Chan, KP, Wang, CC, Chu, CY, Li, WY, et al. (2010). Green Tea Catechins and Their Oxidative Protection in the Rat Eye, *J Agric Food Chem*, 58 (3): 1523.

226 Chen, L, Yang, X, Jiao, H, Zhao, B. (2003). Tea catechins protect against lead-induced ROS formation, mitochondrial dysfunction, and calcium dysregulation in PC12 cells. *Chem Res Toxicol,* Sep;16(9):1155-61.

227 Sinha, D, Roy, S, Roy, M. (2010). Antioxidant potential of tea reduces arsenite induced oxidative stress in Swiss albino mice. *Food Chem Toxicol,* Apr;48(4):1032-9.

228 Ibid. Cia. (2014).

229 Ibid. Landrum. (1997).

230 Ibid. Feher. (2005).

231 Zhang, X, Tohari, AM, Marcheggiani, F, Zhou, X, Reilly, J, et al. (2017). Therapeutic potential of co-enzyme Q10 in retinal diseases. *Curr Med Chem,* Aug 1.

232Littarru, GP, Tiano, L. (2007). Bioenergetic and antioxidant properties of coenzyme Q10: recent developments. *Mol Biotechnol,* Sep;37(1):31-7.

233 Feher J, Kovacs, B, Kovcs, I, Schveoller, M, Papale, A, et al. (2005). Improvement of visual functions and fundus alterations in early age-related macular degeneration treated with a combination of acetyl-L-carnitine, n-3 fatty acids, and coenzyme Q10. *Ophthalmologica,* May-Jun;219(3):154-66.

234Feher, J, Papale, A, Mannino, G, Gualdi, Balacco, GC, et al. (2003). Mitotropic compounds for the treatment of age-related macular degeneration. The metabolic approach and a pilot study. *Ophthalmology,* Sep-Oct;217(5):351-7.

235Ibid. Feher. (2003).

236 Zhang, X, Tohari, AM, Marcheggianai, F, Zhou, X, Reilly, J, et al. (2017). Therapeutic potential of co-enzyme Q10 in retinal diseases. *Curr Med Chem,* 2017;24(39):4329-4339.

237 Bucheli, P, Vidal, K, Shen, L, Gu, Z, Zhang, C, et al. (2011). Goji berry effects on macular characteristics and plasma antioxidant levels, *Optom Vis Sci,* Feb;88(2):257-62.

[238] Tsang, NC, Penfold, PL, Snitch, PJ, Billson, F. (1992). Serum levels of antioxidants and age-related maculardegeneration. *Doc Ophthalmol*, 81(4):387-400.

[239] Mayer, MJ, van Kuijk, FJ, Ward, B, Glucs, A. (1998). Whole blood selenium in exudative age-related maculopathy. *Acta Ophthalmol Scand*, Feb;76(1):62-7.

[240] Ghosh, S, Saha, M, Das, D. (2013). A study on plasma homocysteine level in age-related macular degeneration. *Nepal J Ophthalmol,* Jul-Dec;5(2):195-200.

[241] Huang, P, Wang, F, Sah, BK, Jiang, J, Ni, Z, et al. (2015). Homocysteine and the risk of age-related macular degeneration: a systematic review and meta-analysis. *Sci Rep*, Jul;21;5:10585.

[242] Ganapathy, PS, Perry, RL, Tawfik, A, Smith, RM, Perry, E, et al. (2011). Homocysteine-mediated modulation of mitochondrial dynamics in retinal ganglion cells. *Invest Ophthalmol Vis Sci*, Jul 25;52(8):5551-8.

[243] Johnson, S. (2001). The multifaceted and widespread pathology of magnesium deficiency. *Med Hypotheses*, Feb;56(2):163-70.

[244]Multicenter ophthalmic and nutritional age-related macular degeneration study--part 1: design, subjects and procedures. Age-related Macular Degeneration Study Group. (1996). *J Am Optom Assoc*, Jan;67(1):12-29.

[245] Benavente-Garcia, O, Castillo, J. (2008). Update on uses and properties of citrus flavonoids: new findings in anticancer, cardiovascular, and anti-inflammatory activity. *J Agric Food Chem.* Aug 13;56(15):6185-205.

[246] Tarasiuk, A, Mosinska, P, Fichna, J. (2018). Triphala: current applications and new perspectives on the treatment of functional gastrointestinal disorders. *Chin Med,* Jul 18;13:39.

[247] Ibid. Tarasiuk. (2018).

[248] Peterson, CT, Denniston, K, Chopra, D. (2017). Therapeutic Uses of Triphala in Ayurvedic Medicine. *J Altern Complement Med,* Aug:23(8):607-614.

[249] Shanmuganathan, S, Angayarkanni, N. (2018). Chebulagic acid, Chebulinic acid and Gallic acid, the active principles of Triphala, inhibit

TNFalpha induced pro-angiogenic and pro-inflammatory activites in retinal capillary endothelial cells by inhibiting p38, ERK and NRkB phosphorylation. *Vascul Pharmacol,* Sep;108:23-35.

[250] Nashine, S Konodia, R, Nesburn, AB, Soman, G, Kuppermann, BD, et al. (2019). Nutraceutical effects of Emblica officinalis in age-related macular degeneration. *Aging (Albany NY).* Feb 28;11(4):1177-1188.

[251] Lu, K, Basu, S. (2015). The natural compound chebulagic acid inhibits vascular endothelial growth factor A mediated regulation of endothelial cell functions. *Sci Rep.* 2015;5:9642.

[252] Lu, K, Chakroborty, D, Sarkar, C, Lu, T, Xie, Z, et al. (2012). Triphala and its active constituent chebulinic acid are natural inhibitors of vascular endothelial growth factor-a mediated angiogenesis. *PLoS One.* 2012;7(8):e43934.

[253] Christen, WG, Glynn, RJ, Chew, EY, Albert, CM, Manson, JE. (2009). Folic Acid, Vitamin B6, and Vitamin B12 in Combination and Age-related Macular Degeneration in a Randomized Trial of Women. *Arch Intern Med,* Feb 23;169(4):335-41.

[254] Huang, P, Wang, F, Sah, BK, Jiang, J, Ni, Z, et al. (2015). Homocysteine and the risk of age-related macular degeneration: a systematic review and meta-analysis. *Sci Rep,* Jul;21;5:10585.

[255] Tan, PL, Rickman, CB, Katsanis, N. (2016). AMD and the alternative complement pathway: genetics and functional implications. *Hum Genomics,* 10: 23

[256] Kauppinen, A, Paterno, JJ, Blasiak, J, Salminen, A, Kaarniranta, K. (2016). Inflammation and its role in age-related macular degeneration, *Cell Mol Life Sci,* 1765–1786.

[257] Cho, E, Seddon, JM, Rosner, B, Willett, WC, Hankinson, SE. (2004). Prospective study of intake of fruits, vegetables, vitamins, and carotenoids and risk of age-related maculopathy. *Arch Ophthalmol,* 122(6):883-892

[258] Wang, JJ, Buitendijk, GH, Rochtchina, E, Lee, KE, Klein, BE, et al. (2014). Genetic susceptibility, dietary antioxidants, and long-term

incidence of age-related macular degeneration in two populations. *Ophthalmology*, Mar;121(3):667-75.

[259] Hogg, R, Chakravarthy, U. (2004). AMD and micronutrient antioxidants. *Curr Eye Res*, Dec;29(6):387-401.

[260] Ibid. Vives-Bauza. (2008).

[261] Ibid. Cho. (2004).

[262] Smith, W, Mitchell, P, Leeder, SR. (2000). Dietary fat and fish intake and age-related maculopathy. *Arch Ophthalmol*, 118(3): 401–404.

[263] SanGiovanni, JP, Chew, EY. (2005). The role of omega-3 long-chain polyunsaturated fatty acids in health and disease of the retina. *Prog Retin Eye Res*, 2005;24(1): 87–138.

[264] Merle, B, Delyfer, MN, Korobelnik, JF, Rougier, MB, Colin, J, et al. (2001). Dietary omega-3 fatty acids and the risk for age-related maculopathy: the Alienor Study. *Invest Ophthalmol Vis Sci*, 2001;52(8): 6004–6011.

[265] Augood, C, Chakravarthy, U, Young, I, Vioque, J, de Jong PT, Bentham G, et al. (2008). Oily fish consumption, dietary docosahexaenoic acid and eicosapentaenoic acid intakes, and associations with neovascular age-related macular degeneration. *Am J Clin Nutr*, 88(2): 398–406.

[266] Merle, BM, Delyfer, MN, Korobelnik, JF, Rougier, MB, Malet, F, et al. (2013). High concentrations of plasma n3 fatty acids are associated with decreased risk for late age-related macular degeneration. *J Nutr*, 143(4): 505–511.

[267] Chong, EW, Kreis, AJ, Wong, TY, Simpson, JA, Guymer, RH. (2008). Dietary omega-3 fatty acid and fish intake in the primary prevention of age-related macular degeneration: a systematic review and meta-analysis. *Arch Ophthalmol*, 126(6): 826–833

[268] Ibid. Chiu. (2007).

[269] Maher TJ, Wurtman R. (1987). Possible neurologic effects of aspartame, a widely used food additive. *J Environ Health Perspect*. Nov; 75():53-57.

[270] Rycerz K, Jaworska-Adamu JE. (2013). Effects of aspartame metabolites on astrocytes and neurons. *Folia Neuropathol.* 51(1):10-17.

[271] Kozisek, Frantisek,Health Risks from Drinking Demineralized water, *National Institute of Public Health Czech Republic* https://www.who.int/water_sanitation_health/dwq/nutrientschap12.pdf

[272] Kruse, J. (2012). Quantum Biology 5: Coherent Water=EZ Water. Retrieved Nov 26 2017 from https://www.jackkruse.com/quantum-biology-5-coherent-water/.

[273] Sherwin, JC, Kokavec, J, Thornton, SN. (2015). Hydration, fluid regulation and the eye: in health and disease. *Clin Exp Ophthalmol,* Nov;43(8):749-64

[274] Andriessen, EM, Wilson, AM, Mawambo, G, Dejda, A, Miloudi, K, et al. (2016). Gut microbiota influences pathological angiogenesis in obesity-driven choroidal neovascularization. *EMBO Mol Med*, Dec 1;8(12):1366-1379.

[275] Rowan, S, Jiang, S, Korem, T, Szymanski, J, Chang, ML, et al.(2017). Involvement of a gut-retina axis in protection against dietary glycemia-induced age-related macular degeneration. *Proceedings of the National Academy of Science, USA*, May:114(22)4472-81.

[276] Age-Related Eye Disease Study Research Group. (2001). A randomized, placebo-controlled, clinical trial of high-dose supplementation with vitamins C and E, beta carotene, and zinc for age-related macular degeneration and vision loss: AREDS report no. 8. *Arch Ophthalmol*, 119(10):1417–1436.

[277] Cho, E, Hung, S, Willett, WC, Spiegelman, D, Rimm, EB, et al. (2001). Prospective study of dietary fat and the risk of age-related macular degeneration. *Am J Clin Nutr*, 73(2): 209–218.

[278] Ibid. Cho. (2001).

[279] Chiu, CJ, Milton, RC, Klein, R, Gensler, G, Taylor, A. (2007). Dietary carbohydrate and the progression of age-related macular degeneration: A prospective study from the Age-Related Eye Disease Study. *Am J Clin Nutr*, 86(4):1210-8.

[280] Feng, J, Chen, X, Sun, X, Wang, F, Sun, X. (2014). Expression of endoplasmic reticulum stress markers GRP78 and CHOP induced by oxidative stress in blue light-mediated damage of A2E-containing retinal pigment epithelium cells. *Ophthalmic Res*, 52(4):224-33.

[281] Tosini, G, Ferguson, I, Tsubota, K. (2016). Effects of blue light on the circadian system and eye physiology. *Mol Vis*, PMC4734149.

[282] Allen, MJ, Jarding, JB, Zelner, R. (1998). Macular Degeneration Treatment with Nutrients and Micro Current Electricity. *J. Orthomol Med*, 13:10-12.

[283] Leland, DM, Allen, MJ. (1993). Nutritional supplementation, electrical stimulation and age related macular degeneration. *J Orthomol Med*, 8:168-171.

[284] Shinoda, K, Imamura, Y, Matsuda, S, Seki, M, Uchida, A, et al. (2008). Transcutaneous Electrical Retinal Stimulation Therapy for Age-Related Macular Degeneration. *Open Ophthalmol J*, 2: 132–136.

[285] Reader, AL, Halloran, G. (1997). Bioelectrical Stimulation in an Integrated Treatment for Macular Degeneration, RP, Glaucoma, CMV, and DR. *Fourth Annual Symposium on Biological Circuits*, Oct. Mankato University, MN.

[286] Wallace, LB. (1997). Treatment for Macular Degeneration Utilizing Micro-Current Stimulation, Journal of Optometric Phototherapy. *J Optom Photo*, March.

[287] Paul, E. (2002). The Treatment of Retinal Disease With MCS and Nutritional Supplementation. *International Society for Low-Vision Research and rehabilitation* at the Low Vision Congress in Gothenberg, Sweden.

[288] O'Clock, GD, Jarding, JB. (2009). Electrotherapeutic device/protocol design considerations for visual disease applications. *Engineering in Medicine and Biology Society*, EMBC 2009. Annual International Conference of the IEEE. 2009:2133-6.

[289] Chaikin, L, Kashiwa, K, Bennet, M, Papastergious, G, Gregory, W. (2015). Microcurrent stimulation in the treatment of dry and wet macular degeneration. *Clin Ophthalmol*, 9: 2345–2353.

[290] Myers, CE, Klein, BE, Gangnon, R, Sivakamaran, TA, Lyengar, SK, et al. (2014). Cigarette smoking and the natural history of age-related macular degeneration: the Beaver Dam Eye Study. *Ophthalmology*, Oct;121(10):1949-55

[291] Liew, G, Mitchell, P, Wong, TY, Rochtchina, E, Wang, JJ. (2013). The association of aspirin use with age-related macular degeneration. *JAMA Intern Med*, Feb 25;173(4):258-64.

[292] Kruse, J. (2013). EMF 5: What are the Effects of EMF? Retrieved Oct 20 2017 from https://www.jackkruse.com/emf-5-what-are-the-biologic-effects-of-emf.

[293] Kim, JH, Yu, DH, Kim, HJ, Huh, YH, Cho, SW, et al. (2017). Exposure to 835 MHz radiofrequency electromagnetic field induces autophagy in hippocampus but not in brain stem of mice. *Toxicol Ind Health*, Jan 1:748233717740066.

[294] D'Angelo, C, Costantini, E, Karnal, MA, Reale, M. (2015). Experimental model for ELF-EMF exposure: Concern for human health. *Saudi J Biol Sci*, Jan;22(1):75-84.

[295] Patruno, A, Tabrez, S, Pesce, M, Shakil, S, Kamal, MA, et al. (2015). Effects of extremely low frequency electromagnetic field (ELF-EMF) on catalase, cytochrome P450 and nitric oxide synthase in erythro-leukemic cells. *Life Sci*, Jan 15;121:117-23.

[296] Kruse, J. (2012). EMF 1: Does Your Rolex Work? Retrieved Nov 28 2017 from www.jackkruse.com/emf-1.

[297] Kondrot, EC. Macular Degeneration and Chelation. Retrieved Nov 28 2017 from http://www.fmpug.com/images/upload_files/Macular%20Degeneration%20and%20Chelation_Kondrot.pdf.

[298] NIH Research News. (2013). Chelation Therapy May Help Reduce Cardiovascular Events. Retrieved Nov 20 2017 from https://www.nih.gov/news-events/nih-research-matters/chelation-therapy-may-help-reduce-cardiovascular-events.

[299] Maniscalco, BS, Taylor, KA. (2004). Calcification in coronary artery disease can be reversed by EDTA-tetracycline long-term chemotherapy. *Pathophysiology*Oct;11(2):95-101.

[300] Undersea & Hyperbaric Medical Society. Retrieved Nov 28 2017 from http://www.uhms.org.

[301] Malerbi, FK, Novais, EA, Emmerson, B, Bonomo, PP, Pereira, AJ. (2015). Hyperbaric oxygen therapy for choroidal neovascularization: a pilot study. *Undersea Hyperb Med,* Mar-Apr;42(2):125-31.

[302] Yonekawa, Y, Hypes, SM, Abbey, AM, Williams, GA, Wolfe, JD. (2016). Exacerbation of macular oedema associated with hyperbaric oxygen therapy. *Clin Exp Oppthalmol,* Sep;44(7):625-626.

[303] Borrelli, E, Bocci, V. (2013). Visual improvement following ozonetherapy in dry age related macular degeneration; a review. *Med Hypothesis Discov Innov Ophthalmol,* Summer;2(2):47-51.

[304] BottomLineInc. Slow Down Macular Degeneration with IV Nutrient Therapy. Retrieved 8/10/2017 from https://bottomline-inc.com/health/macular-degeneration/slow-down-macular-degeneration-with-iv-nutrient-therapy.

[305] Gemenetzi, M, Lotery, AJ. (2014). The role of epigenetics in age-related macular degeneration. Eye,Dec; 28(12): 1407–1417

[306] Wei, L, Chen, P, Lee, JH, Nussenblatt. (2014). Genetic and Epigenetic Regulation in Age-related Macular Degeneration. *Asia Pac J Ophthalmol (Phila),* July-August; 2(4): 269–274.

[307] Levin, D. (2015). New Approach to Treating Macular Degeneration. Retrieved May 2 2018 from http://now.tufts.edu/articles/new-approach-treating-macular-degeneration.

[308] Ratnayake, K, Payton, JL, Lakmal, OH, Karunarathne, A. (2018). Blue light excited retinal intercepts cellular signaling. *Sci Rep,* Jul 5;8:10207

Other Books by Safe Goods

The Shattered Oak	$ 14.95
A Barnstormer Aviator	$ 12.95
Flying Above the Glass Ceiling	$ 14.95
Spirit & Creator (Spirit of St. Louis)	$ 29.95
Letters from My Son	$ 22.95
Nutritional Leverage for Great Golf	$ 9.95
Overcoming Senior Moments Expanded	$ 9.95
Prevent Cancer, Strokes, Heart Attacks	$ 11.95
Cancer Disarmed Expanded	$ 7.95
Eye Care Naturally	$ 8.95
Velvet Antler	$ 9.95

www.SafeGoodsPublishing.com